T0269168

SpringerBriefs in Statistics

More information about this series at http://www.springer.com/series/8921

Mikhail Nikulin · Hong-Dar Isaac Wu

The Cox Model and Its Applications

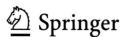 Springer

Mikhail Nikulin
Université Bordeaux Segale
Bordeaux
France

Hong-Dar Isaac Wu
National Chung-Hsing University
Taichung
Taiwan

ISSN 2191-544X
SpringerBriefs in Statistics
ISBN 978-3-662-49331-1
DOI 10.1007/978-3-662-49332-8

ISSN 2191-5458 (electronic)

ISBN 978-3-662-49332-8 (eBook)

Library of Congress Control Number: 2016935392

Printed on acid-free paper

This Springer imprint is published by Springer Nature
The registered company is Springer-Verlag GmbH Berlin Heidelberg

To our families

Preface

Since Sir David Cox's pioneering work in 1972, the proportional hazards (PH) model has become the most important model in survival analysis and in related applications. The success of the Cox model stimulated further studies in semiparametric and nonparametric theory, counting process models, study designs in epidemiology, and the development of many other regression models which could be more flexible or reasonable in data analysis. Flexible semiparametric regression models are used increasingly often in carcinogenesis studies to relate lifetime distributions to time-dependent explanatory variables. In addition to classical regression models such as the Cox PH model and the accelerated failure time (AFT) model, alternative models like the linear transformation model, the frailty model, and some varying-effect models are also considered by researchers (Martinussen and Scheike 2006; Scheike 2006; Dabrowska 2005, 2006; Bagdonavičius 1978; Zeng and Lin 2007). In this monograph, we discuss some important parametric models as well as several semiparametric regression models. Several classical examples are reconsidered and analyzed here, including the well-known datasets concerning effects of chemotherapy and chemo- plus radiotherapy on the survival of gastric and lung cancer patients (Stablein and Koutrouvelis 1985; Piantadosi 1997; Kalbfleisch and Prentice 2002; Klein and Moeschberger 2003). Following the lines of Scheike (2006), Zeng and Lin (2007), Wu (2007), Huber et al. (2006), we also give examples to illustrate and compare possible applications of the Cox model (1972), the Hsieh model (2001), and Bagdonavicius and Nikulin (2002); Bagdonavičius and Nikulin (2005, 2006) simple cross-effect (SCE) model. All three of them are particularly useful to analyze survival data with one crossing point. This monograph offers a short course or one-semester material for undergraduate or graduate students, for biostatisticians, and for scientific researchers who demand applications of survival analysis and reliability theory in areas such as gerontology, demography, insurance, clinical trials, medicine, epidemiology, and social sciences.

Bordeaux, France   Mikhail Nikulin
Taichung, Taiwan   Hong-Dar Isaac Wu
March 2014

References

Bagdonavičius, V. (1978). Testing the hyphothesis of the additive accumulation of damages. *Probability Theory and its Applications, 23*(2), 403–408.

Bagdonavicius, V., & Nikulin, M. (2002). Goodness-of-fit tests for accelerated life models. In Huber, N. Balakrishnan, M. Nikulin & M. Mesbah (Eds.), *Goodness-of-fit tests and model validity* (pp. 281–300). Birkhauser: Boston.

Bagdonavičius, V., & Nikulin, M. (2005). Analyse of survival data with non-proportional hazards and crossing of survival functions. In L. Edler & C. Kitsos (Eds.), *Quantitative methods in cancer and human health risk assessment* (pp. 197–209). New York: Wiley.

Bagdonavičius, V., & Nikulin, M. (2006). On goodness-of-fit for homogeneity and proportional hazards. *Applied Stochastic Models in Business and Industry, 22*, 607–619.

Dabrowska, D. (2005). Quantile regression in transformation models. *Sankhya, 67*, 153–187.

Dabrowska, D. (2006). *Estimation in a class of semi-parametric trasformation models*. In J. Rojo (Ed.), *Second Eric L. Lehmann symposium—Optimality* (pp. 131–169). Institute of Mathematical, Statistics, Lecture Notes and Monograph Series, 49.

Huber, C., Solev, V., & Vonta, F. (2006). Estimation of density for arbitrarily censored and truncated data. In M. Nikulin, D. Commenges & C. Huber (Eds.), *Probability, statistics and modelling in public health* (pp. 246–265). New York: Springer.

Kalbfleisch, J. D., & Prentice, R. L. (2002). *The statistical analysis of failure time data* (2nd ed.). New York: Wiley.

Klein, J. P., & Moeschberger, M. L. (2003). *Survival analysis* (2nd ed.). New York: Springer.

Martinussen, T., & Scheike, T. (2006). *Dynamic regression models for survival functions*. Springer: New York.

Piantadosi, S. (1997). *Clinical trials*. New York: Wiley.

Scheike, T. H. (2006). A flexible semiparametric transformation model for survival data. *Lifetime Data Analysis, 12*, 461–480.

Stablein, D. M., & Koutrouvelis, I. A. (1985). A two sample test sensitive to crossing hazards in uncensored and singly censored data. *Biometrics, 41*, 643–652.

Wu, H.-D. I. (2007). A partial score test for difference among heterogeneous populations. *Journal of Statistical Planning and Inference, 137*, 527–537.

Zeng, D., & Lin, D.Y. (2007). Maximum likelihood estimation in semiparametric regression models with censored data. *Journal of the Royal Statistical Society: Series B, 69*, 509–564.

Acknowledgments

We are deeply grateful for the support, help, discussions, and nice papers of our friends and colleagues, C. Huber, Z. Ying, F. Hsieh, V. Bagdonavicius, V. Solev, W. Meeker, N. Limnios, M.L.T. Lee, S. Gross, N. Singpurwalla, F. Vonta, W. Kahle, H. Lauter, U. Jensen, A. Lehmann, D. Dabrowska, M. Mesbah, N. Balakrishan, W. Nelson, V. Couallier, and L. Gerville-Reache. They introduced us to different branches of survival analysis and the theory of reliability. Our interest for this research fields was boosted with the appearance of the books of Sir Cox and Oakes (1984), Andersen et al. (1993), Lawless (2003), Meeker and Escobar (1998), Martinussen and Scheike (2006), and Hougaard (2000). Finally we would like to thank all our friends and our families.

References

Andersen, P. K., Borgan, O., Gill, R., & Keiding, N. (1993). *Statistical models based on counting processes*. New York: Springer.
Cox, D. R., & Oakes, D. (1984). *Analysis of survival data*. London: Chapman and Hall.
Hougaard, P. (2000). *Analysis of multivariate survival data*. New York: Springer.
Lawless, J. F. (2003). *Statistical models and methods for lifetime data*. New York: Wiley.
Martinussen, T., & Scheike, T. (2006). *Dynamic regression models for survival functions*. New York: Springer.
Meeker, W. Q., & Escobar L., (1998), *Statistical methods for reliability data*. Wiley.

Contents

1 Introduction: Several Classical Data Examples for Survival Analysis.   1
  1.1   Example 1: The Standford Heart Transplant (SHT) Data.   2
  1.2   Example 2: Length of Hospital Stay of Rehabilitating Stroke Patients in Taiwan   4
  1.3   Example 3: Gastric Carcinoma Data.   4
  1.4   Example 4: The Veteran's Administration Lung Cancer Trials. . . .   6
  1.5   Example 5: Other Lung Cancer Data from a Clinical Trial   7

2 Elements of Survival Analysis.   9
  2.1   Basic Concepts, Notations, and Classical Models. 10
  2.2   Classical Parametric Models for Complete Data. 12
  2.3   Censored Data. 20
  2.4   Doob–Meyer Decomposition 22
  2.5   Nelson–Aalen Estimator 23
  2.6   Kaplan–Meier Estimator 23
  2.7   Covariates or Stresses. 25
  2.8   Accelerated Life Models. 26
  2.9   Step-Stresses 26
  2.10 Transformation of the Time Under Covariates 29

3 The Cox Proportional Hazards Model 35
  3.1   Some Properties of the Cox Model on E_1 37
        3.1.1   Tampered Failure Time Model 38
        3.1.2   Model GM 39
  3.2   Some Simple Examples of Alternatives for the PH Models 41
  3.3   Partial Likelihood Estimation 43
        3.3.1   Breslow Estimator for the Baseline Cumulative Hazard Function. 44
        3.3.2   The Stanford Heart Transplant Data as an Example 45

3.4   Log-Rank Test and Robust Tests for Treatment Effect   46
       3.4.1   Log-Rank Test and Weighted Log-Rank Test   46
       3.4.2   Robust Inference: Preliminary   47
       3.4.3   Robust Test with Covariates Adjustment   48

4   **The AFT, GPH, LT, Frailty, and GLPH Models**   53
    4.1   AFT Model   53
    4.2   The GPH Models   57
    4.3   The GPH Models with Monotone Hazard Ratios   59
    4.4   The Second GPH Model   60
    4.5   The GLPH Model   61

5   **Cross-Effect Models of Survival Functions**   63
    5.1   Change Point Model   64
    5.2   Parametric Weibull Regression with Heteroscedastic
           Shape Parameter   64
    5.3   Cox-Type Model with Varying Coefficients   65
    5.4   Hsieh Model   66
           5.4.1   Estimating Equation Processes   68
           5.4.2   Sieve Approximation   69

6   **The Simple Cross-Effect Model**   71
    6.1   Semiparametric Estimation   74
    6.2   An Iterative Procedure for Computing the Estimators   76
    6.3   Analysis of Gastric Cancer Data   77
    6.4   Multiple Cross-Effects Model   78

7   **Goodness-of-Fit for the Cox Model**   81
    7.1   Omnibus Tests   82
           7.1.1   Gill–Schumacher Test   82
           7.1.2   Lin Test   83
    7.2   Test for PH Assumption Within a Wider Class   84
           7.2.1   The GPH and SCE Models as Alternative Hypothesis   84
           7.2.2   The Hsieh Model as an Alternative   87
    7.3   Test for Homogeneity Within a Wider Class: Two-Sample
           Problem   88
           7.3.1   GPH and SCE Models   88
           7.3.2   The Hsieh Model   90
           7.3.3   Examples   93
    7.4   Goodness-of-Fit for the Cox Model from Left Truncated
           and Right-Censored Data   96
           7.4.1   Examples   99

**8   Remarks on Computations in Parametric and Semiparametric
       Estimation**   101

9   Cox Model for Degradation and Failure Time Data   109
      9.1   Aging and Longevity, Failure and Degradation   109
      9.2   Joint Model   112

References   115

Index   121

Chapter 1
Introduction: Several Classical Data Examples for Survival Analysis

The proportional hazards (PH) model was proposed by Sir David Cox just over 40 years ago (Cox 1972). Today, the Cox model is the most important model in survival analysis, reliability and quality of life research, epidemiology, clinical trials, and biomedical studies. There have also been tremendous applications of the Cox model in demography, econometrics, finance, pharmacology, biology, gerontology, insurance, etc. These have marked the great success of the Cox PH model which further induced extended studies of competitive survival regression models and the corresponding development of semiparametric estimation theory, likelihood principle, counting process modeling and applications.

The developments in reliability and survival analysis have provided the basis and useful methods to obtain general theory. A patient's survival depends on his/her age, sex, fatigue, genetic or physiological damages, the dynamics of body temperature, body weight (or BMI), some physiological or biochemical indices, and also on the presence of chronic disease (like cancer, diabetes mellitus, renal disease, cardiac disease, metabolic syndrome, etc.). In general, these characteristics are coded as the so-called *covariates* or *explanatory variables*; some of them are called degradation processes. We suppose that the *lifespan* of an individual is described by *covariates*. In this case, the survival (or failure) of a patient is characterized by this covariate process and by the random moment of its potential failures. The Cox model is an example which relates the lifetime distributions to a set of covariates by modeling hazard rate.

The popularity and the success of the Cox model is based on the fact that there exist simple semiparametric estimation procedures and that the regression parameter in the PH model is easily interpreted as (log-) hazard ratio. The hazard ratios under different fixed covariates are usually assumed to be constant in time. In practice, the hazard rates may approach, go away from, or even intersect each other. In these circumstances, using the conventional Cox PH model to estimate the hazard ratio leads to biased inference. The phenomenon of *nonproportionality* may be derived from several aspects: First, some authors have considered the heterogeneity effect coming from individuals with unobserved frailty so that extra variations may be present (Hougaard 1984, 1986; Aalen 1988). Second, nonproportionality is part

© The Author(s) 2016
M. Nikulin and H.-D.I. Wu, *The Cox Model and Its Applications*,
SpringerBriefs in Statistics, DOI 10.1007/978-3-662-49332-8_1

of the result of the time-varying effect, which could possibly be modeled by the *varying coefficient* Cox model (Martinussen and Scheike 2006). Third, the interaction between time and a qualitative covariate gives nonproportionality (O'Quigley 1991). Finally, some observable covariates contribute both to the mean and to the variance of the lifetime variable or its transformation (Bagdonavičius and Nikulin 1999; Hsieh 2001; Zeng and Lin 2007), and thus produce "nonproportional hazards." In the last case, stratification by some variables can eliminate part of the nonproportionality. However, stratification is not reasonable if a variable is of continuous type and, in particular, when the sample size is not large. Nevertheless, the Cox model helps to construct dynamic models well adapted to the study of survival functions with cross-effect. The PH model is generalized by assuming that at any moment, the hazard ratio depends on time-varying covariates. Relations with generalized proportional hazards, frailty, linear transformation, Sedyakin and degradation models and cross-effect models have been considered. Using some new flexible regression models, in this monograph, we analyze survival data of the Gastrointestinal Tumor Study Group (Stablein and Koutrouvelis 1985), the Veteran's Administration lung cancer trials, the data of Piantadosi (1997) on lung cancer patients, the Stanford Heart Transplant data, and a dataset concerning the length of hospital stay of rehabilitating stroke patients.

These data examples illustrate the characteristics of survival data which may be collected from clinical operation (the Standford Heart Transplant data), hospital registration system (length of hospital stay for stroke patients), and clinical trials (gastric cancer data and lung cancer data). In these data, survival estimates using the Kaplan–Meier method (see Chap. 2) are presented when the characteristics of proportional hazards (see Chap. 3) or nonproportional hazards (see Chaps. 5 and 6) according to different covariate configurations are considered.

1.1 Example 1: The Standford Heart Transplant (SHT) Data

The SHT data reported in Miller and Halpern (1982) contains 184 patients with the following variables: survival time, dead/alive status, age and T5 mismatch scores. Cox and Oakes (1984, Chap. 8) tabulated another version of the SHT data which comprises 249 patients with transplant indicators and waiting times. Here, we consider the data presented in Miller and Halpern (1982). A complete dataset with 154 observations is used. We display the Kaplan–Meier (KM) survival estimates for different age and mismatch score groups. Derivation of the KM estimate and its properties are discussed in Chap. 2.

For the 154 observed times, 102 failured and 52 "right-censored" (explained in Chap. 2) times, the three quartiles of age are 35.0, 44.5, and 49.0. The younger two groups (age $\leq$ 35.0 and 35 $<$ age $<$ 45) have no statistical difference in the lifetimes using the log-rank test (see Chap. 3); these two groups are combined. So we divide the patients into three groups: "age $<$ 45," "45 $\leq$ age $\leq$ 49," and "age $\geq$ 50." The survival estimates are shown in Fig. 1.1(a). The mismatch score measures the tissue incompatibility between recipient and donor; it can be viewed as a continuous random variable. The log-rank test reveals no significant difference in the lifetime distributions among the four groups formed by the quartiles 0.69, 1.05, and 1.49. We simply use the *median* (T5 = 1.05) as the cut-off point and plot the KM estimates for the two groups (Fig. 1.1b).

These two figures show that the survivals are significantly different in age, but not in (dichotomized) mismatch score. The group "age $\geq$ 50" has a sudden drop in survival at the early stage (time $<$ 100 days). The other two younger groups have crossings at an early stage and at a time very close to 2000 days. It appears that the "difference between groups" varies with time. With a proportional hazards regression setting (Chap. 3), the effect of age cannot be modeled by a simple *univariate* variable age. As indicated by this example, seeking an alternative model is important.

Fig. 1.1 a KM estimates for different age groups. **b** KM estimates for different mismatch score groups. Reprinted from Journal of Statistical Planning and Inference, 139(12), H.-D.I. Wu, F. Hsieh, Heterogeneity and Varying Effect in Hazards Regression, pp. 4213–4222, Copyright 2015, with permission from Elsevier

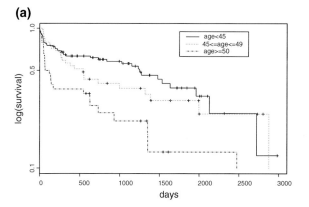

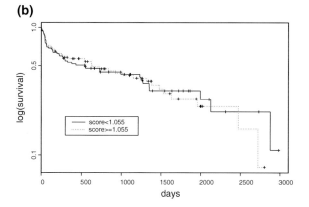

1.2   Example 2: Length of Hospital Stay of Rehabilitating Stroke Patients in Taiwan

Cerebral vascular disease was among the leading causes of death in Taiwan in recent decades (crude mortalities, 53.5–78.4 cases per 10^5 person-years), and rehabilitating stroke patients often had a long length of hospital stay (LOS). The work of study of the principal factors affecting LOS is essential for the management of health-care costs, of after-discharge home care, and of bed occupancy in hospitals of different levels, etc. Further, LOS is a factor related to short-term prognosis and is also an indicator of long-term survival of patients. These data offer an example for the case of *non-censoring* (see Chap. 2); that is, the time of "discharge" from hospital is treated as an "event time." The data enrolled 586 patients who experienced their first hemorrhage/infarct strokes and received in-hospital rehabilitations (Lin et al. 2009). The baseline data include age, gender, co-morbidity status, and previous history of stroke and/or severe injury, etc. Modified Barthel index (MBI) and functional independence measure (FIM) questionnaires were administrated to patients admitted for rehabilitation. The MBI and FIM are two different scores measuring the severity of disability and functional dependence/independence level of patients. These two scores are highly correlated and both indicative of a patient's discharge. In this data, 24.6, 60.8, and 14.6 % of the patients had MBI $= 0$, $0 <$ MBI ≤ 30, and MBI $\geq$ 35; and 24.4, 48.0, and 27.6 % had FIM between [18,28], [29,63] and [64, 125], respectively.

The KM "survival" estimates for different MBI and FIM groups are displayed in Fig. 1.2. Different Barthel index groups (upper panel, Fig. 1.2a) and different FIM groups (lower panel, Fig. 1.2b) both have the proportional hazards relationship. In Lin et al. (2009), confidence intervals of mean LOS are constructed based on the PH model assumption.

1.3   Example 3: Gastric Carcinoma Data

When analyzing survival data from *clinical trials, cross-effects of survival functions* are sometimes observed. A classical example is the well-known data concerning effects of *chemotherapy (CH)* and *chemotherapy plus radiotherapy (CH+R)* on the survival times of *gastric cancer* patients studied by Stablein and Koutrouvelis (1985). The number of patients is 90. Survival times of chemotherapy (group 0 of size 45) and chemotherapy plus radiotherapy (group 1 of size 45) patients are as follows (* denotes right-censored observations). For further details and discussions, see also Kleinbaum and Klein (2005), Klein and Moeschberger (2003), Bagdonavičius et al. (2002), Hsieh (2001), Bagdonavičius et al. (2004), and Zeng and Lin (2007).

Fig. 1.2 **a** KM estimates for different BAR (or MBI) groups. **b** KM estimates for different FIM groups. Reprinted from Journal of the Formosan Medical Association, 108(8), C.-L. Lin, P.-H. Lin, L.-W. Chou, S.-J. Lan, N.-H. Meng, S.-F. Lo, H.-D.I. Wu, Model-based Prediction of Length of Stay for Rehabilitating Stroke Patients, pp. 653–662, Copyright 2015, with permission from Elsevier

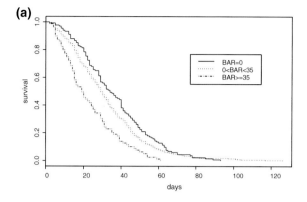

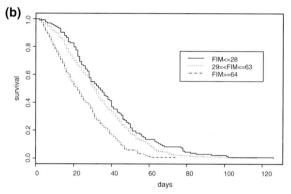

- *Chemotherapy*: 1 63 105 129 182 216 250 262 301 301 342 354 356 358 380 383 383 388 394 408 460 489 499 523 524 535 562 569 675 676 748 778 786 797 955 968 1000 1245 1271 1420 1551 1694 2363 2754* 2950*;
- *Chemotherapy plus Radiotherapy*: 17 42 44 48 60 72 74 95 103 108 122 144 167 170 183 185 193 195 197 208 234 235 254 307 315 401 445 464 484 528 542 567 577 580 795 855 1366 1577 2060 2412* 2486* 2796* 2802* 2934* 2988*.

At the beginning of treatment, the mortality of *CH+R* patients is greater but at a certain moment the survival functions of *CH+R* and *CH* patients intersect, and later the mortality of *CH* patients is greater. That is, if patients survive *CH+R* therapy during a certain period then later this treatment is more beneficial than the *CH* therapy. Doses of *CH* and *R* therapy can be different so regression data can be collected. One will observe (Fig. 1.3) this "cross-effect" phenomena by plotting the *Kaplan–Meier* estimators of the survival function for both treatment groups. The two estimated curves indicate that *radiotherapy* would initially be detrimental to a patient's survival but become beneficial later on. We shall consider models for analysis of data with cross-effect of survival functions under *constant covariates* in

Fig. 1.3 KM estimates for gastric cancer data

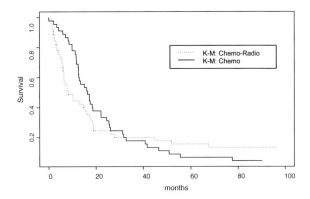

Chaps. 5 and 6. Moreover, we show in Chap. 7 that the conventional log-rank test has low power in this example. The results will be compared between a class of weighted log-rank tests and a score test based on a more flexible model.

1.4   Example 4: The Veteran's Administration Lung Cancer Trials

We studied the survival data of 137 *lung cancer* patients given in Kalbfleisch and Prentice (2002), Bennett (1983), Kleinbaum and Klein (2005), Marubini and Valsecchi (1995), and Therneau and Grambsch (2000), concerning the *Veteran's Administration Lung Cancer Trials*. The dataset includes the following variables: survival time and (right-) censoring status, performance status (Karnofsky rating), cell type of carcinoma (squamous cell, small cell, adeno, and large cell), treatment indicator, months from diagnosis, age, and prior therapy. For ease of illustration, we analyze the *influence of performance status* (Karnofsky rating: 10–30 completely hospitalized, 40–60 partial confinement, 70–90 able to care for self) on the survivals. The *Karnofsky index* is often used to measure the general health status (*degradation*) of a patient (Karnofsky and Burchenal 1949). There are 22 (16.1 %), 57 (41.6 %), and 58 (42.3 %) persons who have the respective Karnofsky ratings (KR): $KR \leq 30, 30 < KR \leq 60,$ and $KR > 60$.

In our example nine observations were censored, i.e., the proportion of censorings is 0.0657. This example illustrates a case when the hazard rates under different values of the covariate do not intersect but the ratios of hazard rates are monotone. That is, the interrelations among these three groups change over time and the proportionalities among the three groups are questionable (Fig. 1.4).

Fig. 1.4 KM estimates for
different Karnofsky indices

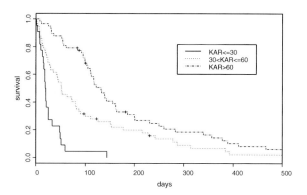

1.5 Example 5: Other Lung Cancer Data from a Clinical Trial

Piantadosi (1997, Chap. 19, pages 483–488) gives the data concerning the survival
times of lung cancer patients. There are 164 patients divided into two groups who
received radiotherapy (sample size 86; Group A) or radiotherapy plus "CAP" (sample size 78; Group B). Apart from survival time and censoring status, the variables include: cell type (67 squamous versus 97 non-squamous), performance status
(abbreviated as PS: there are 20 "PS = 1" and 144 "PS = 2"), tumor status (abbreviated as TS: there are 19 "TS = 1," 92 "TS = 2" and 53 "TS = 3"), nodal status
(NS: 15 "NS = 0," 30 "NS = 1" and 119 "NS = 2"), disease-free survival, indicator
for recurrence, age, race (24 others and 140 whites), weight loss (WL: 142 "WL =
0" and 16 "WL = 1"; 6 missings), and sex (47 females and 117 males). The variable age has quartiles 52.0 (Q1), 58.0 (Q2) and 64.5 (Q3) with sample mean 57.4.
Dichotomizing "age" by a its Q2 leads to nonsignificant difference in the lifetime
distributions (p-value = 0.536, log-rank test). These data exhibit a nonproportional
hazards pattern in treatment, cell type, tumor status, nodal status, weight loss, and

Fig. 1.5 KM estimates for
lung cancer data. Reprinted
from Wiley Books 2nd edn,
S. Piantadosi, Clinical Trials:
A Methodologic Perspective,
p. 125, Copyright 2015, with
permission from Wiley

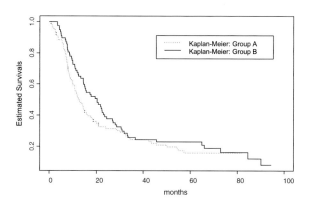

the dichotomized age groups. No significant comparison results can be found in all the above variables using the log-rank test. For illustration, the K–M survival estimates for the two treatments are plotted in Fig. 1.5, in which the K–M estimates cross at 33 months, and the common survival of these two groups is 0.26. We show in Chap. 7 how this data (K–M survivals) can be fitted by two flexible regression models, the Hsieh model and the simple cross-effect model. For the disease-free survivals, proportional hazards assumption seems reasonable and conventional PH analysis applies.

Chapter 2
Elements of Survival Analysis

Failures of highly reliable units are rare. In order to obtain a complementary reliability information, the *accelerated life testing* (ALT) is used so that *higher level of experimental factors* are applied to obtain failures quickly. Alternatively, complementary reliability information can be obtained by measuring some parameters which characterize the *aging, wear or degradation of the product on time*.

Statistical inference from ALT is possible if **failure time regression models** are *well chosen*. The regression models relate failure time distributions to *internal* and *external* explanatory variables (covariates, stresses) influencing the reliability. Before using complex models in any analysis, we suggest that the *Cox's proportional hazards (PH) model* (Cox 1972 1975; Cox and Oakes 1984) can be tried first to give simple results.

In case the data suggest that proportionality can be questionable, practitioners seek to use alternative models. Selection of the candidate model depends on (i) the deviations between data and the estimated PH model and (ii) the feasibility and interpretation of the model. We suppose that the following data are available for reliability characteristics estimation: failure times (possibly *censored*), *explanatory variables* (covariates, stresses), and the values of some observable quantity characterizing the degradation of units. Moreover, the failure rate of a unit is assumed to depend on *covariates, degradation level, and time*. For more details about this, see, for examples, Nelson (1990), Andersen et al. (1993), Klein and Moeschberger (2003), Aven and Jensen (1999), Meeker and Escobar (1998), Hsieh (2001), Lawless (2003), Bagdonavičius and Nikulin (2002a), Ceci and Mazliak (2004), Dabrowska (2005–2007), Martinussen and Scheike (2006), Huber et al. (2006, 2008), Nikulin and Wu (2006), Zeng and Lin (2007), Lehmann (2004), Kahle and Wendt (2006), Bagdonavicius et al. (2011), Voinov et al. (2013).

© The Author(s) 2016
M. Nikulin and H.-D.I. Wu, *The Cox Model and Its Applications*,
SpringerBriefs in Statistics, DOI 10.1007/978-3-662-49332-8_2

2.1 Basic Concepts, Notations, and Classical Models

Let the positive random variable T denotes the failure time of a patient (unit). The probability of a unit functioning up to time t is given by the *survival function* or *reliability function* $S(\cdot)$:

$$S(t) = \mathbf{P}\{T > t\}, \quad t > 0. \tag{2.1}$$

The function $F(t) = 1 - S(t)$ is called the *cumulative distribution function* (cdf) of the lifetime T, and $f(t) = dF(t)/dt$ is the probability density when T is continuous.

In reliability and survival analysis, the *hazard rate* function $\lambda(\cdot)$ of *the lifetime T* is defined as

$$\lambda(t) = \lim_{h \to 0} \frac{1}{h} \mathbf{P}\{t \leq T < t + h | T \geq t\} = -\frac{d[\ln S(t)]}{dt}, \quad t > 0. \tag{2.2}$$

The hazard rate specifies the *instantaneous rate of mortality* or *failure* at time t. It follows that $\lambda(t) = f(t)/S(t)$ and

$$S(t) = e^{-\Lambda(t)}, \tag{2.3}$$

where $\Lambda(t) = \int_0^t \lambda(s)ds (t > 0)$ is the *cumulative hazard function* of the failure time T. It is evident from (2.3) that $\Lambda(\cdot)$ is an *increasing function* with $\Lambda(0) = 0$ and $\Lambda(\infty) = \infty$.

The deterministic function $\Lambda(t)$ is also called the *natural degradation process* of the population. The population disappears when $\Lambda(t)$ reaches *the infinity*.

The models discussed in survival analysis and reliability theory are often formulated in terms of cumulative hazard and hazard rate functions. The most common shapes of hazard rates are *monotone*, ∪-*shaped*, or ∩-*shaped*, See, for example, Meeker and Escobar (1998). For more details on the use of classical *parametric models*, one can refer to Cox and Oakes (1984), Kalbfleisch and Prentice (2002), Lawless (2003), Bagdonavičius et al. (2011).

Figure 2.1 is the plot of two hazard functions of Weibull distributions with different parameter conditions producing monotone increasing and monotone decreasing hazards. The corresponding cumulative hazard and survival functions are plotted in Figs. 2.2 and 2.3. We illustrate in these figures how the three functions (hazard, cumulative hazard, and survival) correspond to one another. From a practical point of view, the application of a *Weibull distribution without modification* is limited because a hazard in Fig. 2.1 is quite large when time approaches to 0; see Sect. 5.2 for more discussions.

Fig. 2.1 $\lambda_{x(\cdot)}(t) = 2t$ and $\lambda_{x_0(\cdot)}(t) = \lambda_0(t) = \frac{1}{2\sqrt{t}}$

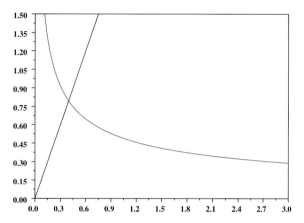

Fig. 2.2 $\Lambda_{x(\cdot)}(t) = t^2$ and $\Lambda_{x_0(\cdot)}(t) = \Lambda_0(t) = \sqrt{t}$

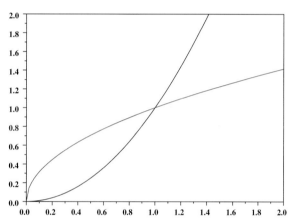

Fig. 2.3 $S_{x(\cdot)}(t) = e^{-t^2}$ and $S_{x_0(\cdot)}(t) = S_0(t) = e^{-\sqrt{t}}$ one can see here the cross-effect of survival functions

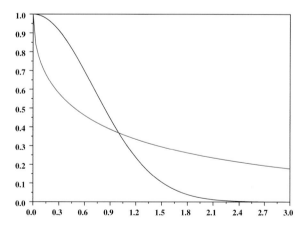

2.2   Classical Parametric Models for Complete Data

Let the positive random variables $T_1, T_2, \ldots, T_n$ be failure times. If the data are complete (not censored), then there are two possibilities to estimate the distribution function (or survival function). First, to construct the *empirical distribution function*

$$F_n(t) = \frac{1}{n} \sum_{i=1}^{n} \mathbf{1}_{(-\infty, t]}(T_i), \quad t \in \mathbf{R}^1,$$

based on the observed simple sample $T_1, T_2, \ldots, T_n$. In survival analysis it is assumed that T_i are positive random variables, $\mathbf{E} T_i < \infty$ and we can write

$$F_n(t) = \frac{1}{n} \sum_{i=1}^{n} \mathbf{1}_{(0, t]}(T_i), \quad t > 0.$$

It is a *nonparametric unbiased estimator* for the distribution function $F(t)$,

$$\mathbf{E} F_n(t) \equiv F(t), \quad t > 0.$$

It follows that $S_n(t) = 1 - F_n(t)$ is a nonparametric unbiased estimator for the survival $S(t)$.

Second, the distribution of T_i can be assumed to belong to a given *parametric* class,

$$\{f(t, \theta), \quad \theta \in \Theta\}.$$

Then we may estimate the unknown parameter θ by its *maximum likelihood estimator* $\hat{\theta}_n$:

$$\hat{\theta}_n = argmax_\theta L(\theta), \quad \theta \in \Theta,$$

where

$$L(\theta) = \prod_{i=1}^{n} f(T_i, \theta), \quad \theta \in \Theta,$$

is *the likelihood function* constructed on the basis of complete data $T_1, T_2, \ldots, T_n$ under the model $f(\cdot, \theta)$. Now we have the parametric estimators $f(t, \hat{\theta}_n), F(t, \hat{\theta}_n)$ and $S(t, \hat{\theta}_n) = 1 - F(t, \hat{\theta}_n)$ for the density, the distribution and survival functions f, F and S respectively. Parametric approach is relatively simple and easy to implement. Statistical analysis of parametric models can be done by a classical manner (Cox and Oakes 1984; Hjort 1992; Meeker and Escobar 1998). The most frequently used parametric distributions include: exponential, Gompertz–Makeham, Weibull, gamma, log-normal, log-logistic, inverse Gaussian, the power Generalized Weibull distributions, exponentiated Weibull families, and hypertabastic distributions, among others. Here we sketch the simple properties of these distributions.

Example 1. Exponential model.

The most simple parametric lifetime model is the exponential model. The hazard rate of an exponential lifetime variable T is *constant in time*:

$$\lambda(t) \equiv \lambda = const > 0,$$

where λ is called the *parameter of intensity of events*. The corresponding survival function of T is

$$S(t) = S(t; \lambda) = \mathbf{P}\{T > t\} = e^{-\lambda t}, \quad t > 0, \tag{2.4}$$

with

$$\mathbf{E}T = \frac{1}{\lambda}, \quad \mathbf{Var}T = \frac{1}{\lambda^2}$$

and the *linear cumulative hazard function*

$$\Lambda(t) = \lambda t, \quad t > 0.$$

From (2.4) it follows that for any t and $s > 0$

$$\mathbf{P}\{T > t + s | T > s\} = \mathbf{P}\{T > t\} = e^{-\lambda t}. \tag{2.5}$$

Equation (2.5) explains why it is called *no aging* or *lack of memory*, simply because λ is a constant.

Example 2. Gompertz–Makeham model.

We have the *Gompertz–Makeham model* if the hazard rate function of the *lifetime T* is given by

$$\lambda(t) = \lambda(t; \alpha, \beta, \gamma) = \beta + \alpha e^{\gamma t}, \quad t > 0, \quad \alpha > 0, \quad \gamma > 0, \quad \beta > 0.$$

This model is particularly useful in the researches of aging in demography, gerontology, pharmacology, and economy.

Example 3. Weibull model.

The *Weibull model* is commonly used in reliability and biomedical areas when the survival function of the lifetime T is written as

$$S(t) = S(t; \nu, \theta) = e^{-(t/\theta)^\nu}, \quad t > 0, \quad \nu > 0, \quad \theta > 0,$$

with the associated hazard rate function

$$\lambda(t) = \lambda(t; \nu, \theta) = \frac{\nu}{\theta^\nu} t^{\nu-1}.$$

The parameters θ and ν are named as the *scale* parameter and *shape* parameter, respectively. It follows that $\lambda(\cdot)$ is monotone *increasing* if $\nu > 1$, *decreasing* if $0 < \nu < 1$, and *constant in time* if $\nu = 1$. It is evident that this model is more flexible than the exponential model.

Example 4. Gamma model.
The lifetime T follows the *gamma distribution* if it has the density function

$$f(t; p, \lambda) = \frac{\lambda^p t^{p-1} e^{-\lambda t}}{\Gamma(p)}, \quad t > 0, \quad p > 0, \quad \lambda > 0,$$

where $\Gamma(p) = \int_0^\infty t^{p-1} e^{-t} dt$, the gamma function. The hazard rate of the gamma model is

$$\lambda(t) = \lambda(t; p, \lambda) = \frac{t^{p-1} e^{-\lambda t}}{\int_t^\infty u^{p-1} e^{-\lambda u} du},$$

where p is the *shape parameter*. It is monotone *increasing* for $p > 1$ and *decreasing* for $0 < p < 1$.

Example 5. Log-normal model.
The *Log-normal* (LN) family of distributions $LN(\mu, \sigma)$ has the survival function

$$S(t) = S(t; \mu, \sigma) = 1 - \Phi\left(\frac{\ln t - \mu}{\sigma}\right), \quad \mu \in R^1, \quad \sigma > 0, \quad t > 0.$$

The hazard function of the LN distribution is *unimodal* and is very popular in modeling fatigue failures in industry.

Example 6. Log-logistic model.
The *log-logistic model* (LL) is also used often in reliability and survival analysis. The lifetime T follows the LL distribution if it has the survival function

$$S(t) = S(t; \theta, \nu) = \frac{1}{1 + (t/\theta)^\nu}, \quad t > 0, \quad \theta > 0, \quad \nu > 0.$$

In this case, the hazard rate function is

$$\lambda(t) = \lambda(t; \theta, \nu) = \frac{\nu}{\theta^\nu} t^{\nu-1} \left[1 + \left(\frac{t}{\theta}\right)^\nu\right]^{-1}, \quad t > 0.$$

If $\nu > 1$, the hazard rate function is *hump shaped* ($\cap$): it *increases* to its *maximum*, and then approaches to 0 *monotonically* as $t \to \infty$.

Example 7. Inverse Gaussian Model.
The lifetime T of the *inverse Gaussian* (IG) distribution has the following pdf:

$$f(t) = f(t; \lambda, \mu) = \sqrt{\frac{\lambda}{2t^3\pi}} \exp\left\{-\frac{\lambda(t-\mu)^2}{2t\mu^2}\right\}, \quad t > 0, \quad \lambda > 0, \quad \mu > 0.$$

It is easy to verify that $\mathbf{E}T = \mu$ and $\mathbf{Var}T = \mu^3/\lambda$. The hazard rate function of T has the $\cap$-*shape*.

Example 8. The Birnbaum–Saunders model.
The family of Birnbaum–Saunders (BS) distributions, proposed by Birnbaum and Saunders (1969), is used when the failures are due to *crack*. This family has two parameters: *shape* parameter and *scale* parameter. *Fatigue failure* is often due to repeated applications of a common *cyclic stress* pattern.

The cumulative distribution function of *two-parameter Birnbaum–Saunders distribution* is

$$F(t) = F(t; \alpha, \beta) = \Phi\left[\frac{1}{\alpha}\left\{\left(\frac{t}{\beta}\right)^{\frac{1}{2}} - \left(\frac{\beta}{t}\right)^{\frac{1}{2}}\right\}\right], \quad t > 0, \quad \alpha, \beta > 0,$$

where α is the *shape parameter*, β is the *scale parameter*, and $\Phi(x)$ is the cdf of standard normal distribution function. The probability density function can be written for $t > 0$ as

$$f(t) = f(t; \alpha, \beta) = \frac{1}{2\sqrt{2\pi}\,\alpha\beta}\left\{\left(\frac{\beta}{t}\right)^{\frac{1}{2}} + \left(\frac{\beta}{t}\right)^{\frac{3}{2}}\right\} \exp\left[-\frac{1}{2\alpha^2}\left(\frac{t}{\beta} + \frac{\beta}{t} - 2\right)\right].$$

The hazard function of this distribution is *unimodal* and is popular in modeling fatigue failures in industry. Other *unimodal* distributions include: *log-normal, inverse Gaussian, log-logistic*, power generalized Weibull, exponentiated Weibull, etc.

Desmond (1986) and Meeker and Escobar (1998) have worked on the relationship between BS distribution and the IG distribution. The hazard functions for both of BS and IG distributions are very similar. We note that the *gamma, log-logistic, log-normal, inverse Gaussian*, and BS distributions are often used for the construction of the so-called *frailty models*, parametric AFT, and Cox models. Extensive works have been done recently on the BS and IG distributions and their applications in the failure time data analysis of *the redundant systems*.

Example 9. Power generalized Weibull model.
The *power generalized Weibull* (PGW) distribution (Bagdonavičius and Nikulin 2002a) has the survival function (of the lifetime T):

$$S(t) = S(t; \gamma, v, \theta) = exp\left\{1 - \left[1 + \left(\frac{t}{\theta}\right)^v\right]^{\frac{1}{\gamma}}\right\}, \quad t > 0, \ \gamma > 0, \ v > 0, \ \theta > 0.$$

If $\gamma = 1$ we have the conventional Weibull family of distributions. If $\gamma = 1$ and $v = 1$, we have the exponential family of distributions. The hazard rate function of T is

$$\lambda(t) = \lambda(t; \gamma, v, \theta) = \frac{v}{\gamma\theta^v}t^{v-1}\left[1 + \left(\frac{t}{\theta}\right)^v\right]^{\frac{1}{\gamma}-1}, \quad t > 0.$$

A significant property of this class of distributions is: all moments of this distribution are finite. The hazard rate has different *shapes* for the following parameter conditions:

1. *constant* (for $v = \gamma = 1$),
2. *monotone increasing* (for $v > 1$, $v > \gamma$ and for $v = 1$, $\gamma < 1$),
3. *monotone decreasing* (for $0 < v < 1$, $v < \gamma$ and for $0 < v < 1$, $v = \gamma$),
4. *unimodal* or $\cap$-*shaped* (for $\gamma > v > 1$), and
5. *bathtub-* or $\cup$-*shaped* for $0 < \gamma < v < 1$.

Note that the last type of shape includes three period: *burn in infant mortality* (or simply *burn in*) period, relatively *low failure intensity period*, and *senility* period with *progressively increasing risk of failure* (which is the period of *aging* and *degradation*).

Finally, we have a remark on the survival function of this distribution. Suppose that $\theta = v = 1$ and let $a = \frac{1}{\gamma} > 0$. Under these conditions, the survival function $S(t) = S_{GW}(t)$ is given by

$$S_{GW}(t) = e^{1-(1+t)^a}, \quad t \geq 0.$$

We want to know the behavior of the survival function $S_{GW}(t)$ near $t = 0$, i.e., when $t \sim 0$.

Note that if $t \sim 0$, then

$$e^{1-(1+t)^a} \asymp 2 - (1+t)^a \asymp 1 - at,$$

from where it follows that if $t \sim 0$ then

$$S_{GW}(t) \asymp 1 - at \quad \text{and} \quad F_{GW}(t) \asymp at$$

under given conditions.

Example 10. Exponentiated Weibull model.
The *exponentiated Weibull (EW) family* of distributions were proposed by Mudholkar and Srivastava (1993) and Mudholkar et al. (1995). The EW distribution has the survival function $S(t)$ and probability density function $f(t)$:

$$S(t) = S(t; \gamma, \nu, \theta) = 1 - \left\{ 1 - exp\left[-\left(\frac{t}{\theta}\right)^{\nu} \right] \right\}^{1/\gamma}, \quad t > 0, \quad \gamma > 0, \quad \nu > 0, \quad \theta > 0.$$

$$f(t) = f(t; \gamma, \nu, \theta) = \frac{\nu}{\gamma\theta} \left\{ 1 - exp\left[-\left(\frac{t}{\theta}\right)^{\nu} \right] \right\}^{\frac{1}{\gamma} - 1} exp\left[-\left(\frac{t}{\theta}\right)^{\nu} \right] \left(\frac{t}{\theta}\right)^{\nu-1}.$$

This model has all properties of the GW model. As claimed by Mudholkar et al. (1995, Theorem 2.1), the hazard function can be monotone increasing ($\nu \geq 1$ and $\nu/\gamma \geq 1$), monotone decreasing ($\nu \leq 1$ and $\nu/\gamma \leq 1$), bathtub-shaped ($\nu > 1$ and $\nu/\gamma < 1$), and unimodal ($\nu < 1$ and $\nu/\gamma > 1$).

We also have a small remark on the survival function of the exponentiated Weibull distribution, assuming $\theta = \nu = 1$ and denoting $a = \frac{1}{\gamma} > 0$, $a \neq 1$. Under these conditions, $S(t) = S_{EW}(t)$ is given by

$$S_{EW}(t) = 1 - [1 - e^{-t}]^a, \quad t \geq 0.$$

Note that if $t \sim 0$, then
$$1 - e^{-t} \asymp 1 - (1 - t) \asymp t,$$

from where it follows that if $t \sim 0$ then

$$S_{EW}(t) \asymp 1 - t^a \quad \text{and} \quad F_{EW}(t) \asymp t^a$$

under given conditions.

Example 11. Hypertabastic model.
The two-parameter family of *Hypertabastic distributions*, $H(\alpha, \beta)$, was recently proposed by Tabatabai et al. (2007). Because $t > 0$, this distribution can be used for different applications in reliability and survival analysis. Tabatabai et al. (2007) proposed to use this parametric model to construct the baseline function in survival models. The hazard rate function can be monotone (increasing or decreasing) or ∩-shape, depending on the parameter values. In particular, for ∩-shape hazard, this distribution is competitive to other distributions such as log-normal, log-logistic, inverse Gaussian, power generalized Weibull, etc.

Let X be a positive random variables. We say that X follows the hypertabastic distribution $H(\alpha, \beta)$ if its cumulative distribution function is

$$F(t, \theta) = 1 - \text{Sech}\left\{ \frac{\alpha}{\beta}\left(1 - t^{\beta} \text{Coth}(t^{\beta})\right) \right\}, \quad t > 0, \quad \theta = (\alpha, \beta)^T \in \mathbf{R}_*^+ \times \mathbf{R}_*^+,$$

where, Sech($\cdot$) and Coth($\cdot$) are hyperbolic secant and hyperbolic cotangent, respectively. Its survival function is

$$S(t, \theta) = \text{Sech}\left\{ \frac{\alpha}{\beta}\left(1 - t^{\beta} \text{Coth}(t^{\beta})\right) \right\}, \quad t > 0, \quad \theta = (\alpha, \beta)^T \in \mathbf{R}_*^+ \times \mathbf{R}_*^+,$$

Hypertabastic probability density and hazard functions are given by the next formulas:

$$f(t, \theta) = \alpha t^{\beta-1}\{t^\beta \mathrm{Csch}^2(t^\beta) - \mathrm{Coth}(t^\beta)\}\, \mathrm{Sech}\{W(t, \theta)\}\mathrm{Tanh}\{W(t, \theta)\},$$

and

$$\lambda(t, \theta) = \alpha t^{\beta-1}\{t^\beta \mathrm{Csch}^2(t^\beta) - \mathrm{Coth}(t^\beta)\}\, \mathrm{Tanh}\{W(t, \theta)\}.$$

respectively, where, $W(t, \theta) = \frac{\alpha}{\beta}\left(1 - t^\beta \mathrm{Coth}(t^\beta)\right)$.

The hypertabastic hazard function has following interesting properties:

- If $0 < \beta \leq 0.25$, then its hazard rate is decreasing from ∞ to 0.
- If $0.25 < \beta \leq 1$, then its hazard rate is unimodal. It increases with time until reaching its maximum and then decreases.
- If $1 < \beta \leq 2$, then the hazard rate is increasing with upward concavity until reaching the inflection point and then continues to increase with downward concavity thereafter.
- If $\beta > 2$, its hazard rate is increasing with upward concavity.

The consideration of the different hazard shapes bring out the different biological mechanisms of disease progression. This is helpful to clinicians, researches, and pharmacologists to keep track of the disease status over time, (for details, see Tabatabai et al. (2007)). In particular, this family is used for analysis of clinical data in cervical cancer research.

Using the properties of hypertabastic hazard function, we can construct the chi-squared goodness-of-fit test based on the Nikulin–Rao–Robson statistics $\mathbf{Y}_n^2$ and on the properties of the maximum likelihood estimator $\hat{\theta}_n$; see, for example, Voinov et al., (2013). ♣

In survival analysis, *semiparametric models* are often considered. A model is called *semiparametric* if it comprises a parametric part and a nonparametric part. In practice, when a semiparametric model is considered to be further simplified, often the *nonparametric* part (if it involves a baseline survival function S_0) is specified to have a simple parametric distribution such as Weibull, generalized Weibull, gamma, log-logistic, etc. Parametric models were studied, for examples, by Meeker and Escobar (1998), Hjort (1992), Lawless (2003), Aven and Jensen (1999), Lehmann (2004), Kahle and Wendt (2006), etc.

Many parametric distributions can be extended to accommodate regression settings. See the parametric example of Cox model discussed in Chap. 3. However, the use of parametric models have its limitations. For example, in many cases, Weibull regression and log-logistic regression models cannot "fit the data" well if the underlying hazard is bump-shaped or bathtub-shaped. This can be easily checked by discretizing some covariates, and the so-called "data fitting" is displayed by comparing the estimated survivals based on the *parametric* model(s) and those obtained from the *nonparametric* Kaplan–Meier estimates (Nikulin and Wu 2006).

If the parametric methods does not give a good solution, people use the power-ful *nonparametric* methods to estimate S, Λ, λ and other characteristics, using all information from the *empirical distribution*. These methods are well developed since 1970s.

Remark: from parametric distributions to regression

Parametric models can be extended to incorporate covariates information so that the modeling is more flexible and powerful. Taking the Weibull distribution as an example, the survival function of the Weibull distribution

$$S(t) = S(t; \nu, \theta) = e^{-(t/\theta)^{\nu}}$$

has two positive parameters θ and ν. For a set of covariates $\mathbf{z} = (z_1, \ldots, z_p)$, $z_0 = 1$, if these two parameters are further modeled as

$$1/\theta = \exp\{\beta'\mathbf{z}\} = \exp\{\beta_0 + \beta_1 z_1 + \cdots + \beta_p z_p\} \text{ and}$$
$$\nu = \exp\{\gamma'\mathbf{z}\} = \exp\{\gamma_0 + \gamma_1 z_1 + \cdots + \gamma_p z_p\},$$

it is a *parametric* example of Hsieh's (2001) *semiparametric* heteroscedastic hazards regression (HHR) model. Two-sample estimation of the HHR model is discussed in Hsieh (1996). If $\gamma_1 = \cdots = \gamma_p = 0$, the HHR model reduces to the conventional proportional hazards (PH) model.

Remark : on the cross-effects of survivals

When analyzing reliability and survival data from accelerated trials, *cross-effects* of hazard rates are sometimes observed. A classical example is the well-known data of the *Gastrointenstinal Tumor Study Group* (Chap. 1, Example 3), concerning *effects of chemotherapy and radiotherapy* on the survival times of *gastric cancer patients*, (Stablein and Koutrouvelis 1985; Klein and Moeschberger 2003). See also Fleming et al. (1980) for two datasets with cross-effects phenomena: an ovarian cancer data and a bile duct cancer data.

   If the hazard rates of two populations *do not cross*, then we can say that *the risk of failure* of one population *is smaller* than that of the second in time interval $[0, \infty)$. In this casse, one population is named *uniformly more reliable* than the other. Such hypothesis is sometimes more interesting to verify than the hypothesis of equality of distributions (the *homogeneity hypothesis*). If, for example, the hypothesis of equal-ity is not true for the two populations receiving *conventional* and *new* treatments, then it is possible that the new treatment population has better results *only* at the beginning of the process. This suggests some alteration (e.g., changing treatment) must be made before the crossing of hazard rates.

2.3 Censored Data

In medical and epidemiological studies, failure times are typically *right censored*. That means a failure time T is observed if $T \leq C, C > 0$ is called the censoring time. Otherwise we only know that $T > C$. In this book, if only "censored" is used, then we mean "right censored." On the contrary, *left censoring* means that the failure time T is observed if $T \geq C$. There are various types of right-censoring mechanism:

(1) If n "subjects" are censored at a prespecified calender time τ, it is called *type I censoring*. In this case, $C = \tau$ for all subjects.
(2) If the study is terminated whenever a specified number r $(r < n)$ of failures have occurred, it is called *type II censoring*. The time of the rth failure is then defined as the censoring time C for all subjects.
(3) If the failure times $T_1, \ldots, T_n$ and the censoring times $C_1, \ldots, C_n$ are mutually independent positive random variables, it is called *independent random censoring*. For example, if several failure modes are possible and interest is focused on one particular failure mode, then the failure of any other mode can be considered as a random censoring.

For randomly right-censored data, denote T_i and C_i as the failure and censoring times of subject i. Let

$$X_i = T_i \wedge C_i, \quad \delta_i = \mathbf{1}_{\{T_i \leq C_i\}} \quad (i = 1, \ldots, n), \tag{2.6}$$

where $a \wedge b = \min(a, b)$ and $\mathbf{1}_A$ is an indicator of the event A. The following data are observed:

$$(X_1, \delta_1), \ldots, (X_n, \delta_n). \tag{2.7}$$

If $\delta_i = 1$, it is known that a *failure* occurs at the time $T_i = X_i$; if $\delta_i = 0$, then the failure occurs after the time X_i; that is, the subject is *censored* by $C_i = X_i$. One can see that the initial sample $(T_1, \ldots, T_n)$ obtained without censoring is different from (2.7).

To describe right-censored data in terms of *counting processes*, let

$$N_i(t) = \mathbf{1}_{\{X_i \leq t, \delta_i = 1\}} = \mathbf{1}_{\{T_i \leq t, T_i \leq C_i\}} \tag{2.8}$$

be the number of failure of the ith person in the interval $[0, t]$, where $\mathbf{1}_A$ denotes the indicator of the event A. It equals to 1 if one failure is *observed* in this interval; otherwise it equals to 0. The *at-risk* process of the ith person is defined as

$$Y_i(t) = \mathbf{1}_{\{X_i \geq t\}}, \quad t \geq 0. \tag{2.9}$$

It equals to 1 when the ith person is still under observation at time $t-$. Furthermore, let

$$N(t) = \sum_{i=1}^{n} N_i(t), \quad t \geq 0,$$

be the total number of failures observed in the interval $[0, t]$ and

$$Y(t) = \sum_{i=1}^{n} Y_i(t), \quad t \geq 0,$$

be the number of subjects *at risk for failure* just prior to the moment t. More precisely, for any t the value $Y(t)$ gives the number of patients who are at risk for failure during a small time interval $(t - \varepsilon, t]$ for an arbitrarily small positive ε, since any unit that fails exactly at time t must be both in the risk set at the failure time and known to be at risk before the failure occurred.

The stochastic processes N and N_i are actually examples of *counting processes*. With this setting, the data can be presented in the form

$$(N_1(t), Y_1(t), t \geq 0), \ldots, (N_n(t), Y_n(t), t \geq 0). \tag{2.10}$$

Indeed, the above two ways ((2.7) and (2.10)) of data presentation are *equivalent*: If (X_i, δ_i) are given then $(N_i(t), Y_i(t)), t \geq 0$, can be found using their definition. Conversely, X_i is the moment of jump of $Y_i(t)$ from 1 to 0. If $N_i(t)$ has a jump at X_i then $X_i = T_i$ and $\delta_i = 1$; if $N_i(t) = 0$ for any $t \geq 0$ then $X_i = C_i$ and $\delta_i = 0$.

The advantage of using data presentation (10) is as follows. The values of

$$\{N_i(s), Y_i(s), \quad 0 \leq s \leq t; \quad i = 1, \ldots, n\}$$

are known as the *history* of failures and censorings up to time t. The notion of "history" is formalized by the concept of *filtration* (Klein and Moeschberger 2003, Therneau and Grambsch 2000, Huber et al. 2006, Andersen et al. 1993, Fleming and Harrington 1991).

Let us denote

$$\mathscr{F}_t = \sigma\{N_i(s), Y_i(s), 0 \leq s \leq t\}$$

as the σ-*algebra* generated by $N_i(s)$ and $Y_i(s)$, $0 \leq s \leq t$. Here $\mathscr{F}_t$ *contains all events* related with failure and censoring processes which occur before t. That is, $\mathscr{F}_t$ is the smallest σ-*algebra* containing all events

$$\{N_i(s) = k, Y_i(s) = l\}, \quad 0 \leq s \leq t; \quad k, l \in \{0, 1\}.$$

It is clear that $\mathscr{F}_s \subset \mathscr{F}_t \subset \mathscr{F}$, for $0 \leq s \leq t$. The family of σ-algebras $\mathbf{F} = \{\mathscr{F}_t, t \geq 0\}$ is called the *filtration* (or *history*) generated by the data.

All trajectories of the *counting processes* N_i and N are right continuous, nondecreasing piecewise constants with jumps of size 1. It is easy and essential to show that they are *submartingales* with respect to the filtration $\mathbf{F}$.

Remark. In survival analysis and reliability theory, statisticians are working in general with *left-truncated* and *right-censored* samples:

$$(X_1, D_1, \delta_1, z_1), \ldots, (X_n, D_n, \delta_n, z_n),$$

where

$$X_i = T_i \wedge C_i, \quad \delta_i = \mathbf{1}_{\{T_i \leq C_i\}},$$

with T_i being the failure times, D_i the truncation times, and C_i the censoring times. The at-risk indicator is set as:

$$Y_i(t) = \mathbf{1}_{\{D_i < t \leq X_i\}} \ Y(t) = \sum_{i=1}^{n} Y_i(t).$$

If the data are only right-censored then take $D_i = 0$; if the data are only left-truncated then take $\delta_i = 1$. The process $N(t)$ shows for any $t > 0$ the number of observes failures in the interval $[0, t]$ and the process $Y(t)$ shows the number of objects which are "at risk" (under observation and nor failed) just prior to time t. It is supposed that survival distributions of all n objects given x_i are absolutely continuous with the survival functions $S_i(t)$ and the hazard rates $\lambda_i(t)$.

It is also supposed that truncation and censoring are noninformative (see Andersen et al. 1993, Huber et al. 2006, Solev 2009, Turnbull 1976) and the multiplicative intensities model is assumed: The compensator of the counting processes N_i with respect to the history of the observed processes is $\int Y_i \lambda_i du$.

2.4 Doob–Meyer Decomposition

Suppose that the failure times $T_1, \ldots, T_n$ are identically distributed and absolutely continuous; and they are independent of the censoring times $C_1, \ldots, C_n$. The unique *compensator* of the counting process $N(t)$ with respect to the filtration $\mathbf{F}$ is

$$A(t) = \int_0^t Y(u) \, d\Lambda(u),$$

where $\Lambda(t) = \int_0^t \lambda(u) \, du$ is the cumulative hazard function of T. It follows that the process

$$M(t) = N(t) - A(t), \quad t \geq 0,$$

is the *martingale* with respect to the filtration **F**, i.e.,

$$\mathbf{E}\{M(t)|\mathscr{F}_s\} = M(s), \quad \text{for} \quad s < t.$$

This property of martingale $M(t)$ means that the expected value of $M(t)$, given its history at time $s < t$, is equal to its value at time s. It implies the so-called *Doob–Meyer decomposition*:

$$N(t) = A(t) + M(t), \quad t > 0, \tag{2.11}$$

with

$$\mathbf{E}N(t) = \mathbf{E} \int_0^t Y(u) \, d\Lambda(u), \tag{2.12}$$

where $\Lambda(u)$ is the cumulative hazard function of T. We may also interpret (2.11) as

$$observation = model + error.$$

2.5 Nelson–Aalen Estimator

The equality (2.11) holds even when the function $\Lambda(\cdot)$ is not continuous. Moreover, (2.12) implies that an *estimator of the cumulative hazard function* can be defined by the *method of moments* as a solution to the integral equation:

$$\widehat{\Lambda}(t) = \int_0^t \frac{dN(u)}{Y(u)} = \sum_{j:\delta_j=1, X_j \le t} \frac{d_j}{n_j}, \tag{2.13}$$

where

$$n_j = Y(X_j) = \sum_{l=1}^n \mathbf{1}_{\{X_l \ge X_j\}}$$

is the number of individuals at risk just prior to X_j, and d_j is the number of tied failures occurred at X_j. When there are no ties, $\widehat{\Lambda}(t) = \sum_j \frac{1}{n_j}$. It is called the *Nelson-Aalen estimator* of the cumulative hazard Λ.

2.6 Kaplan–Meier Estimator

The survival function $S(t) = \exp\{-\Lambda(t)\}$ of T_i, on one hand, can be estimated as $\widehat{S(t)} = \exp\{-\widehat{\Lambda}(t)\}$. On the other hand, when d_j/n_j is small,

$$\widetilde{S(t)} = \exp\{-\widehat{\Lambda}(t)\} = \exp\left\{-\sum_{j:\delta_j=1,X_j\le t}\frac{d_j}{n_j}\right\} \approx \prod_{j:\delta_j=1,X_j\le t}\left(1-\frac{d_j}{n_j}\right),$$

which suggests an alternative estimator:

$$\widehat{S}(t) = \prod_{j:\delta_j=1,X_j\le t}\left(1-\frac{d_j}{n_j}\right).$$

To derive the above formula more *exactly*, an approach through the product of conditional probabilities can be used. That is, for T_i (or X_i whenever $\delta_i = 1$),

$$S(t_i) = \frac{S(t_i)}{S(t_{i-1})}\cdot\frac{S(t_{i-1})}{S(t_{i-2})}\cdots\frac{S(t_1)}{S(t_0)}\cdot S(t_0),$$

where t_i is the realization of T_i with $t_0 = 0$ and $S(t_0) = 1$. It implies

$$S(t_i) = \mathbf{P}\{T > t_i | T > t_{i-1}\}\mathbf{P}\{T > t_{i-1} | T > t_{i-2}\}\dots\mathbf{P}\{T > t_1 | T > t_0\}$$

$$= \prod_{j:t_j<t_i,\delta_j=1}\left(1-\frac{d_j}{n_j}\right).$$

By counting process notations, $\Delta N(t) = N(t) - N(t-)$ is the number of failures occurred precisely at time t. A conventional form for the survival estimate is expressed as

$$\widehat{S}(t) = \prod_{s:s\le t}\left(1-\frac{\Delta N(s)}{Y(s)}\right). \tag{2.14}$$

It is the nonparametric *Kaplan–Meier estimator* for the survivor function $S(t)$. If there are *tied* failures and $T_1^0 < \cdots < T_m^0$ are the distinct, observed failure times, d_i is the number of failures at the moment T_i^0 and $n_i = Y(T_i^0)$ is the number of subjects *at risk* just prior to T_i^0, then the Kaplan–Meier estimator for $S(t)$ (with tied failures) is

$$\widehat{S}(t) = \prod_{i:T_i^0\le t}\left(1-\frac{d_i}{n_i}\right) \tag{2.15}$$

with a companion estimator for the cumulative hazard:

$$\widehat{\Lambda}(t) = \sum_{i:T_i^0\le t}\frac{d_i}{n_i}.$$

The effects of *tied* observations on statistical inference have been studied by Breslow (1974). It is also known that the Kaplan–Meier estimator is the nonparametric maximum likelihood estimator of the survival function, taken among all piecewise-constant survivals with jumps at the observed failure times.

2.7 Covariates or Stresses

In reliability and survival analysis, the *survival* or *longevity* depends on individual characteristics of units/subjects. In general, these characteristics are expressed as a set of *explanatory variables* (also called *stresses* or *covariates*), which are possibly *time-dependent*. When we consider a class of *flexible* or *accelerated life regression models*, the lifetime distributions are then related to the covariates. These models should be *well adapted* to work with censored data.

The *lifespan* of an unit is appropriate to be described in terms of covariates and some of them are called *degradation processes*. It is evident that covariates can be *internal* and *external*. We suppose that any explanatory variable is given in terms of *deterministic* time function

$$x(\cdot) = (x_1(\cdot), \ldots, x_m(\cdot))^T : [0, \infty[\to R^m, \quad x(\cdot) \in E,$$

where E is a set of all *possible* or *admissible* stresses and $x_i(\cdot)$ are scalar functions. On any set E of admissible stresses, we may consider a class of survival functions, $\{S_{x(\cdot)}(\cdot), x(\cdot) \in E\}$, which could be very rich and considered as being *well adapted* to treat the data

$$(X_i, \delta_i, x^{(i)}(t), 0 \leq t \leq \tau), \quad x^{(i)} \in E, \quad (i = 1, 2, \ldots, n),$$

to give the interesting answers on questions posed by data about our population, etc.

For any stress $x(\cdot) \in E$, it is important to compare the behavior of population under the condition $x(\cdot)$ with the one under the so-called *ideal, standard or normal* condition x_0. The main question is: how to connect $S_{x(\cdot)}$ with S_{x_0}?

Let $z(\cdot)$ and $y(\cdot)$ be two *admissible* stresses: $z(\cdot), y(\cdot) \in E$. We want to ask if the stress $z(\cdot)$ is *accelerated* with respect to the stress $y(\cdot)$. It is known that $z(\cdot)$ is *accelerated* with respect to the stress $y(\cdot)$, if

$$S_{z(\cdot)}(t) \leq S_{y(\cdot)}(t), \quad \forall t \geq 0, \quad S_{z(\cdot)}(\cdot), S_{y(\cdot)}(\cdot) \in \{S_{x(\cdot)}(\cdot), x(\cdot) \in E\}.$$

2.8 Accelerated Life Models

In reliability theory and in the analysis of clinical trials, an important task is to quantify the prediction of survival and longevity, and to control or improve the efficiency of different technology and procedures if covariate information can be well utilized. In many circumstances, the *accelerated life models* can be used to link the lifetimes and the covariates.

The term "accelerated life" is used since the change in the value of stress leads to the change in life condition of an item (or a patient). As a consequence, the changes may *increase* or *decrease* the risk of failure and hence all evolution processes of the population go more quickly or more slowly. By this sense, we say that the individual item or patient experiences an accelerated life.

Note that to construct the accelerated life models, first, we have to determine the impact covariates, and then to understand by which manner they *influence* the survivals. That is to say, the accelerated life models take into account the lifespan and the conditions of subject simultaneously.

2.9 Step-Stresses

Suppose that n items are observed, and the i-th item is tested under the stress $x^{(i)}(\cdot)$. Let the failures be independently right censored so we have the following form of *right-censored data with covariates*:

$$(X_i, \delta_i, x^{(i)}(t), 0 \le t \le \tau), \quad (i = 1, 2, \ldots, n), \tag{2.16}$$

where τ is the *finite time* of the experiment. Let E be the set of all possible (admissible) stresses. If $x(\cdot) \in E$ is *constant in time* we denote x instead of $x(\cdot)$, and E_1 is the set of all admissible (possible) constant covariates, $E_1 \subset E$. The mostly used time-varying stresses in accelerated trials are the *step-stresses*. If there are several units placed on test at an initial low stress and they do *not fail* at a predetermined time t_1, the stress is then *increased*. If they still do not fail at a predetermined time $t_2 > t_1$, the stress *increased* once more, and so on. The *step-stresses* with k steps have the form:

$$x(u) = \begin{cases} x_1, & 0 \le u < t_1, \\ x_2, & t_1 \le u < t_2, \\ \ldots & \ldots \\ x_k, & t_{k-1} \le u < t_k, \quad t_k \le \infty, \end{cases} \tag{2.17}$$

where $x_1, \ldots, x_k$ are from E_1. The sets of *all possible step-stresses* with the form (2.17) are denoted by E_k, $E_k \subset E$. If $k = 2$, for example, then E_2 is a set of *step-stresses* of the form

Fig. 2.4 Increasing
step-stress for the warm
stand-by unit

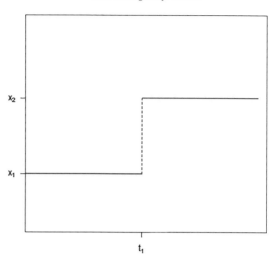

$$x(t) = x_1 \mathbf{1}_{\{0 \le t < t_1\}} + x_2 \mathbf{1}_{\{t_1 \le t\}}, \quad x_1, x_2 \in E_1. \tag{2.18}$$

In most cases, an individual's nature characterizes his/her lifespan. The so-called *characteristic* is represented by a covariate value. If a set of covariates are *well chosen*, the difference in their values and configurations significantly differentiate the survivals between the patients (individuals) (Figs. 2.4, 2.5, 2.6 and 2.7).

Remark. On classification of stresses.
In accelerated life testing, the most used types of stresses are (see Nelson 1990):

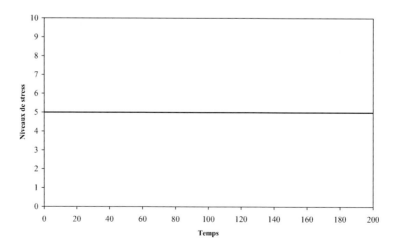

Fig. 2.5 Stress $x = 5$ is a constant in time, $x \in E_1, \quad m = 1$

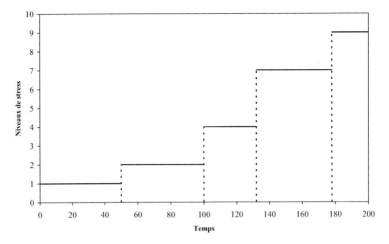

Fig. 2.6 Stress x is an increasing step stress, $x \in E_5$, $m = 1$

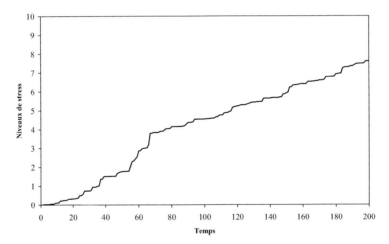

Fig. 2.7 Degradation process

1. *Constant in time stress.*
2. *Step-stress*: a specimen is subjected to successively higher levels of stress. At first, it is subjected to a specified constant stress for a specified length of time. If it does not fail, it is subjected to a higher stress level for a specified time, and so on.
3. *Progressive stress*: a specimen undergoes a continuously increasing level of stress. The most common case—Linearly increasing stress.
4. *Cyclic stress.*
5. *Random stress.*

The most common case is when the stress is unidimensional, for example high temperature, voltage, but more then one accelerating stresses may be used.

In survival analysis the covariate x is a vector, components of which correspond to various characteristics influencing lifetime of individuals such as methods of cure or operation, quantities or types of remedies, environment, interior characteristics as blood pressure, sex, etc. These factors can be as constant as nonconstant in time.

2.10   Transformation of the Time Under Covariates

It can be expected that the survivals and hazard rate functions depend on the covariates as well as on the data *history*. If the history of one patient is described by the deterministic covariate $x(\cdot)$, $x(\cdot) \in E$, and $T = T_{x(\cdot)}$ is the *time-to-failure* under the stress $x(\cdot)$, then the *survival* and *cumulative distribution functions* are

$$S_{x(\cdot)}(t) = \mathbf{P}\left\{T \geq t \mid x(s) : 0 \leq s \leq t\right\}, \quad t \geq 0,$$

and

$$F_{x(\cdot)}(t) = \mathbf{P}\left\{T < t \mid x(s) : 0 \leq s \leq t\right\}, \quad t \geq 0, \tag{2.19}$$

respectively. The *hazard rate function* under $x(\cdot)$ is

$$\lambda_{x(\cdot)}(t) = \lim_{h \downarrow 0} \frac{1}{h} \mathbf{P}\{T_{x(\cdot)} \in [t, t+h) | T_{x(\cdot)} \geq t\} = -\frac{S'_{x(\cdot)}(t)}{S_{x(\cdot)}(t)}, \quad t \geq 0,$$

and the *cumulative hazards function* is

$$\Lambda_{x(\cdot)}(t) = \int_0^t \lambda_{x(\cdot)}(u)du = -\ln\left\{S_{x(\cdot)}(t)\right\}, \quad x(\cdot) \in E, \quad t \geq 0.$$

From these expressions, one can see the dependence of these functions on the life-history *up to time* t. If the explanatory variable is a random process $X(t), t > 0$, and $T_{X(\cdot)}$ is the nonnegative failure time under $X(\cdot)$ then we denote by

$$S_{x(\cdot)}(t) = \mathbf{P}\{T_{X(\cdot)} \geq t | X(s) = x(s), 0 \leq s \leq t\},$$

$$\lambda_{x(\cdot)}(t) = -\frac{S'_{x(\cdot)}(t)}{S_{x(\cdot)}(t)} \quad \text{and} \quad \Lambda_{x(\cdot)}(t) = -\ln\left\{S_{x(\cdot)}(t)\right\}$$

the conditional survival, hazard rate, and cumulative hazard functions, respectively. The definition of "models" should be understood in terms of these conditional functions.

The time-to-failure $T = T_{x(\cdot)}$ could be called the *resource* of the item; the item failed since its resource was used. But the notion of resource should not depend on $x(\cdot)$. Let us consider the *Smirnov's transformation* of the time-to-failure $T = T_{x(\cdot)}$:

$$R = \Lambda_{x(\cdot)}(T_{x(\cdot)}),$$

where $\Lambda_{x(\cdot)}(\cdot)$ is the cumulative hazard rate of T under stress $x(\cdot)$. It is easy to verify that under any $x(\cdot)$ the statistic R has the *standard exponential distribution* with the survival function $S_R(\cdot)$:

$$S_R(t) = \mathbf{P}\{R \geq t\} = e^{-t}, \quad t \geq 0, \quad x(\cdot) \in E, \tag{2.20}$$

in which there is no phenomena of *aging*. Statistic R takes values in the interval $[0, \infty)$ and does not depend on $x(\cdot)$. In a sense, we can say that the standard exponential distribution plays the same role in survival analysis and reliability as the *uniform* distribution on $[0, 1]$ in the theory of probability. We also note that

$$T_{x(\cdot)} = t \quad \text{if and only if} \quad R = \Lambda_{x(\cdot)}(t).$$

For all $x(\cdot)$, the moment t for items working under the stress $x(\cdot)$ is equivalent to the moment $\Lambda_{x(\cdot)}(t)$ for items working in conditions when the time-to-failure has the standard exponential distribution. So the number $\Lambda_{x(\cdot)}(t) \in [0, \infty)$ is called *the exponential resource used until the moment t under the stress $x(\cdot)$*. The concrete item which failed at the moment t under the stress $x(\cdot)$ used $\Lambda_{x(\cdot)}(t)$ of the resource until this moment.

Instead of the exponential resource a statistician can define a resource with any probability distribution, so we can consider a whole class of resource. Suppose that G is the same fixed survival function, strictly decreasing and continuous on $[0, \infty)$ and $H = G^{-1}$ is the inverse function of G. The survival function of the random variable

$$R^G = f_{x(\cdot)}^G(T_{x(\cdot)}) = H(S_{x(\cdot)}(T_{x(\cdot)})), \quad x(\cdot) \in E, \tag{2.21}$$

is G and does not depend on $x(\cdot)$. The statistic R^G is called the *G-resource* and the number $f_{x(\cdot)}^G(T_{x(\cdot)})$ is called the *G-resource used till the moment t*.

In the particular case, when $G = S_{x_0}$ is the survival function under the *normal, standard, or usual stress* x_0 the moment t under the stress $x(\cdot)$ is equivalent to the moment $f_{x(\cdot)}^{S_{x_0}}(t)$ under the normal stress x_0 for all $x(\cdot) \in E$.

Denote $\lambda_{x_0(\cdot)}(\cdot)$ the hazards rate function under the so-called *standard stress* $x_0(\cdot)$. It is the mortality rate under the *normal* conditions corresponding to a stress $x_0(\cdot) \in E$. We shall use the notations S_{x_0} and Λ_{x_0} for the survival and cumulative hazards functions of T under $x_0(\cdot)$. Often $x_0 = x_0(\cdot)$ denotes a *constant* stress.

In order to organize a more informative and efficient comparison for clinical trials done under different covariates and treatments, for example, one have to consider which model is more suitable to the endpoint analysis. In some situations, the main interest of clinicians is to *translate* (or *link*) the p-values between trials. The *equipercentile equating method* (based on equating the p-values) gives a possibility of making decision about the homogeneity or heterogeneity between groups of patients, or about the effectiveness of two considered treatments, etc. In survival analysis, reliability, psychology, and health related quality-of-life researches, this method provides possibilities of incorporating different covariates and using the so-called flexible regression models which are suitable for the analysis under *dynamic* environments. See, for example, Bagdonavicius (1978), Bagdonavicius and Nikulin (1994, 1995, 1998), Kolen and Brennan (2004), Martinussen and Scheike (2006).

A test system with time $f_{x(\cdot)}^{S_{x_0}}(t)$ under the *normal stress* $x_0 = x_0(\cdot)$ is said to be *equivalent* to another system with time t under the stress $x(\cdot)$, if the probability that a unit used under the stress $x(\cdot)$ would survive till the moment t is equal to the probability that a unit used under the stress x_0 would survive till the moment $f_{x(\cdot)}(t)$. That is,

$$S_{x(\cdot)}(t) = \mathbf{P}\{T > t | x(s) : 0 \le s \le t\}$$
$$= \mathbf{P}\{T > f_{x(\cdot)}(t) | x_0(s) : 0 \le s \le f_{x(\cdot)}(t)\} = S_{x_0}(f_{x(\cdot)}(t)), \qquad (2.22)$$

in which for any time t and any stress $x(\cdot) \in E$ we have

$$f_{x(\cdot)}(t) = f_{x(\cdot)}^{S_{x_0}}(t) = S_{x_0}^{-1}\left(S_{x(\cdot)}(t)\right), \quad x(\cdot) \in E. \qquad (2.23)$$

The Eqs. (2.22) and (2.23) show that to construct one family (model) $\{S_{x(\cdot)}, x \in E\}$ we may apply the baseline survival function S_{x_0} and the *transferable* (*linking*) functional (Fig. 2.8)

$$f_{x(\cdot)}(\cdot) : E \times [0, \infty) \to [0, \infty).$$

The value $f_{x(\cdot)}(t)$ is called the *resource used till the moment t* under the stress $x(\cdot)$.

Fig. 2.8 Transfer functional

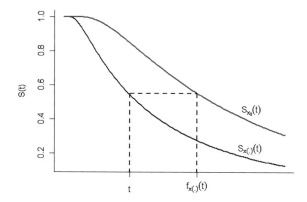

In more general case, we suppose that G is an arbitrary survival function on $[0, \infty)$, such that $G^{-1} = H$ exists. For any covariate $x(\cdot)$ from E at any moment t, we may compare the values $G(t)$ and $S_{x(\cdot)}(t)$ by equating $S_{x(\cdot)}$ and G as

$$S_{x(\cdot)}(t) = G(f_{x(\cdot)}(t)), \tag{2.24}$$

with $f_{x(\cdot)}(0) = 0$, and $S_{x(\cdot)}(t) = \mathbf{P}\{T_{x(\cdot)} \geq t\}$. We obtain the *equipercentile equation*

$$f_{x(\cdot)}(t) = f_{x(\cdot)}^G(t) = G^{-1}\left(S_{x(\cdot)}(t)\right) = H\left(S_{x(\cdot)}(t)\right), x(\cdot) \in E. \tag{2.25}$$

The functional $f_{x(\cdot)}(t) : E \times [0, \infty) \to [0, \infty)$ is called the *transfer functional* (Bagdonavicius and Nikulin 1995) or the *equipercentile transfer functional* (El Fassi et al. 2009).

It is evident that the equipercentile functional is monotone increasing in t for any fixed $x(\cdot)$, and

$$f_{x(\cdot)}(t) \to \infty, \quad \text{when} \quad t \to \infty.$$

The survival function of the statistic

$$R^G = G^{-1}\left(S_{x(\cdot)}(T_x(\cdot))\right) = H\left(S_{x(\cdot)}(T_{x(\cdot)})\right) = f_{x(\cdot)}^G(T_{x(\cdot)}) \tag{2.26}$$

is G and does not depend on $x(\cdot)$. The random variable R^G is called the *G-resource* ($S_{x_0(\cdot)}$-*resource*) or simply the *resource*, and the number $f_{x(\cdot)}^G(t)$ is called the *G-resource used until time t under the stress* $x(\cdot)$. It represents the effect of covariate on the *lifespan*. *Accelerated life* or *flexible* models can be formulated by the specification of resource usage, or more exactly in terms of the *rate of resource using* at any time t:

$$\frac{\partial f_{x(\cdot)}(t)}{\partial t}, \quad x(\cdot) \in E. \tag{2.27}$$

The models of accelerated life will be formulated in dependence on the way of resource using. Note that different resource can have different way of using. This is the cause of considering a whole class of resources. For more about the model construction in accelerated experiments, see Bagdonavičius and Nikulin (1995, 2001a, b)

Example (AFT model). Suppose that for a given family $\{S_{x(\cdot)}, x(\cdot) \in E\}$ there exist a positive survival function G on $[0, +\infty)$ having $H = G^{-1}$ and a positive function $r : E \to R^1$ such that for any $x(\cdot) \in E$

$$S_{x(\cdot)}(t) = G\left(\int_0^t r[x(s)]\, ds\right), \quad x(\cdot) \in E. \tag{2.28}$$

From (2.26) and (2.28) it follows that the G-resource and the G-resource used till the moment t under stress $x(\cdot)$ are

$$R = R^G = \int_0^{T_{x(\cdot)}} r(x(s))ds \quad \text{and} \quad f_{x(\cdot)}^G(t) = \int_0^t r(x(s))ds. \qquad (2.29)$$

Taking derivative of $f_{x(\cdot)}^G(t)$ with respect to t, we obtain the AFT model on E in terms of the G-resource by the next formula:

$$\frac{\partial f_{x(\cdot)}(t)}{\partial t} = r(x(t)), \quad \text{with} \quad f_{x(\cdot)}(0) = 0.$$

That is, the rate of G-resource using at any time t depends only on the value $x(t)$ of the stress $x(\cdot)$ at this moment t, then this family represents the famous *AFT model*. From (2.25) and under the AFT model, any survival function $S_{x(\cdot)}$ from a considered family is expressed in terms of the baseline survival function G and r by (2.28).

The AFT model is widely used and studied in accelerated trails. It can be considered as parametric, semiparametric, or nonparametric. For parametric models used in accelerated life testing, see Meeker and Escobar (1998), Bagdonavicius and Nikulin (2001), Bagdonavicius et al. (2002), Mann et al. (1974), etc. In this case, the function G is taken from some class of distributions as Generalized Weibull, Weibull, log-normal, log-logistic, etc. Semiparametric analysis of AFT model when r is parametrized was considered by Bagdonavicius and Nikulin (1998, 2001), Ying (1993), Shaked and Singpurwalla (1983), etc. Nonparametric estimation when r is not parametrized was considered by Bagdonavicius and Nikulin (1997, 1998, 2000).

The AFT model is also known as the *Additive Accumulation of Damage model*, (AAD), which was proposed by Bagdonavicius (1978). See also Cox and Oakes (1984).

Bagdonavicius and Nikulin (1994, 1995, 1998, 2001) proposed several classes of accelerated life models with time-dependent stresses in terms of resource usage rate (2.27). These models can be practically used if a concrete form of the functional $f_{x(\cdot)}(\cdot)$ is assumed, that is, if an accelerated life model relating failure time to stress is given.

Before our elucidation on the Cox PH model in the next section, it is worth noting that conventional survival models (including the proportional hazards model) do not design the "dynamic" modeling automatically in model formulation. To some extent, *dynamics* means that some covariate(s) has different "effect" at different times. This may induce a consideration of varying-coefficient Cox model (Martinussen and Scheike 2006). On the other hand, "dynamics" may originate from an intrinsic mechanism; which is modeled through an adequate description on the "data history." In epidemiologic studies, however, it is not always possible to capture all covariates that have dynamic influence; and, it is not possible that one can foresee which covariate(s) possess a dynamic effect, or a *cumulative* (or *summing*) effect. In such cases, modeling the hazard rates (at time t) through a set of covariates as well as through the *cumulative hazards just before time t* ($t-$) is a natural consideration. In the sequel, we also discuss several models that have a "dynamic" meaning.

Chapter 3
The Cox Proportional Hazards Model

The *proportional hazards* (PH) or *Cox model* holds on E, if the hazard rate has the form

$$\lambda_{x(\cdot)}(t) = r\{x(t)\}\,\lambda_0(t), \quad x(\cdot) \in E, \tag{3.1}$$

where $\lambda_0(\cdot)$ is an unspecified *baseline hazard rate* function, and $r(\cdot)$ is a positive function on E. The function $r(\cdot)$ explains the *summing effect* of all $x_i(\cdot)$ on the distribution of T. If r is unknown it is a *nonparametric model*. In most applications the function r is parameterized in the form

$$r(x) = \exp\{\beta^T x\},$$

where $\beta = (\beta_1, \ldots, \beta_m)^T$ is the vector of *regression parameters*. Under this parameterization we obtain the classical *semiparametric* Cox model on E with time-dependent covariables:

$$\lambda_{x(\cdot)}(t) = e^{\beta^T x(t)}\lambda_0(t), \quad x(\cdot) \in E. \tag{3.2}$$

If $\lambda_0(\cdot)$ is further taken from some parametric family of hazard rates (the Weibull family, for example), then we have a parametric model. The following example illustrates that the *parametric* Weibull family fulfills the setting of Cox model with covariates.

Example: Parametric example of Cox's model
Consider a class of Weibull distributions indexed by a set of covariates $\mathbf{X} = (X_1, \ldots, X_p)^T$: let $T_{\mathbf{X}}$ be distributed as Weibull with survival function

$$S_{T_{\mathbf{X}}}(t) = \mathbf{P}\{T_{\mathbf{X}} \geq t\} = \exp(-a_* t^b).$$

© The Author(s) 2016
M. Nikulin and H.-D.I. Wu, *The Cox Model and Its Applications*,
SpringerBriefs in Statistics, DOI 10.1007/978-3-662-49332-8_3

Here the scale parameter a_* is modeled as $\exp(\beta_0 + \beta^T \mathbf{X})$ with

$$\beta^T \mathbf{X} = \beta_1 X_1 + \cdots + \beta_p X_p.$$

Then the cumulative hazard

$$\Lambda_{T_\mathbf{X}}(t) = \exp(\beta^T \mathbf{X})(at^b)$$

for $a = \exp(\beta_0)$. By this expression, the Weibull family has the structure of Cox PH model: $\lambda(t; \mathbf{X}) = \lambda_0(t) \exp(\beta^T \mathbf{X})$ if the baseline hazard $\lambda_0(t)$ equals to abt^{b-1} (or the baseline cumulative hazard $\Lambda_0(t) = at^b$). An example for the analysis of Stanford Heart Transplant (SHT) data using Weibull regression is presented in Sect. 3.5 to compare with the estimation of Cox model.

Note that in this example the shape parameter b is a fixed and unknown positive constant. If it is further modeled as $b = \exp(\gamma^T \mathbf{X})$ for a set of parameters $\gamma = (\gamma_1, \ldots, \gamma_p)^T$, then we have the so-called *heteroscedastic hazards regression* (HHR) model proposed by Hsieh (2001). See Sect. 5.4 for further details.   ♣

The PH model is mostly applied for analysis of survival data but the statisticians working in reliability are very cautious to use it, especially for analysis of accelerated life testing data. It can be explained by the fact that the PH model has one unnatural property: the conditional probability to fail in a time interval $(t, t + s)$ given that a unit is functioning at the moment t depends only on the values of the stress (or covariable) $x(\cdot)$ in that interval but does not depend on the values of the stress until the moment t:

$$\mathbf{P}(T \le t + s \mid T > t) = 1 - \exp\left\{-\int_t^{t+s} e^{\beta^T x(u)} d\Lambda_0(u)\right\},$$

here T is failure time, λ_0 is the baseline hazard function which does not depend on stress. For this reason we can say that PH model has the property of *absence of memory*.

The common sense says that if a unit functioned in high stress conditions, it used a large amount of resource and is *"older"* than a unit which functioned in *mild* stress conditions at the same time t. So the conditional probabilities of failure after the moment t should be different for those two units. More exactly, the proportional hazards model suppose that the ratio of resource using at the moment t depends only on values of covariates at this moment and does not depend on resources used until this moment.

Let x_1 and x_2 be two *constant* stresses, $x_1, x_2 \in E_1$, and $x(\cdot) \in E_2$ is a *simple step stress* of the form

$$x(t) = \begin{cases} x_1, & \text{if } t < t_1 \\ x_2, & \text{if } t \ge t_1, \end{cases} \tag{3.3}$$

then for all $t \geq t_1$

$$\lambda_{x(\cdot)}(t) = \lambda_{x_2}(t).$$

If x_1 is some *accelerated stress* with respect to the "*normal*" stress x_2, the resource $\Lambda_{x(\cdot)}(t_1)$ used until the moment t_1 under the stress $x(\cdot)$ is larger than the resource used till the moment t_1 under the stress x_2. Nevertheless, the proportional hazards model states that the rate of resource using is the same after the moment t_1. If, for example, individuals are *aging*, it is not very natural. The hazard rate of individuals who used more of the resource would be higher after the moment t_1. So we need a generalization of the model which includes dependence of the rate of resource using on the *used resource*.

Nevertheless, in survival analysis the PH model usually works quite well, because the values of covariates under which estimation of survival is needed are in the range of covariate values used in experiments. In epidemiologic studies, *cumulative effect* of some variable(s) up to moment t can be naturally created in case the *data history* is known.

So, using a simple model (which could be *not very exact*) often is preferable than using a more complicated model. The case is similar to the classical linear regression models: the mean of the dependent variable is rarely a linear function of the independent variables but the linear approximation works reasonably well in some range of independent variable values.

3.1 Some Properties of the Cox Model on E_1

From (3.1), $\lambda_x(t) = r(x) \lambda_0(t)$, $x \in E_1$, it follows that for any constant in time stress $x \in E_1$ the corresponding survival function S_x has the form :

$$S_x(t) = S_0^{r(x)}(t) = \exp\{-r(x)\Lambda_0(t)\}, \quad x \in E_1,$$

where

$$S_0(t) = e^{-\Lambda_0(t)}$$

and

$$\Lambda_0(t) = \int_0^t \lambda_0(s)ds$$

are the baseline survival and cumulative hazards functions.

It is evident that

$$\Lambda_0(t) = -\ln S_0(t),$$

and for any x

$$\Lambda_x(t) = -\ln S_x(t), \quad x \in E_1.$$

Note that for any $x_0 \in E_1$ the Cox model implies

$$\lambda_x(t) = \rho(x_0, x)\lambda_{x_0}(t), \quad \Lambda_x(t) = \rho(x_0, x)\Lambda_{x_0}(t)$$

and

$$S_x(t) = S_{x_0}^{\rho(x_0, x)}(t),$$

where

$$\rho(x_0, x) = \frac{r(x)}{r(x_0)}.$$

Under the PH model on E_1, the hazard ratio $HR(t, x_0, x)$ between different covariates x and x_0 is constant over time:

$$HR(t, x_0, x) = \rho(x_0, x).$$

From the definition of the PH model on E, we have

$$\Lambda_{x(\cdot)}(t) = \int_0^t r(x(u))d\Lambda_0(u)$$

and

$$S_{x(\cdot)}(t) = \exp\left\{-\int_0^t r(x(u))d\Lambda_0(u)\right\}.$$

3.1.1   Tampered Failure Time Model

Now we are able to give several important properties of PH model for simple step-stresses $x(\cdot) \in E_2$.

Let $x(\cdot)$ has the form given by (3.3). Then it is easy to show that under PH model for any $x(\cdot) \in E_2$

$$\lambda_{x(\cdot)}(t) = \begin{cases} \lambda_{x_1}(t), & 0 \le t < t_1, \\ \lambda_{x_2}(t), & t \ge t_1, \end{cases}$$

$$= \begin{cases} r(x_1)\lambda_0(t), & 0 \le t < t_1, \\ r(x_2)\lambda_0(t), & t \ge t_1. \end{cases}$$

From this, for any $x_0 \in E_1$, we have

$$\lambda_{x(\cdot)}(t) = \begin{cases} \rho(x_0, x_1)\lambda_{x_0}(t), & 0 \le t < t_1 \\ \rho(x_0, x_2)\lambda_{x_0}(t), & t \ge t_1. \end{cases}$$

Taking $x_0 = x_1$ we also have

$$\lambda_{x(\cdot)}(t) = \begin{cases} \lambda_{x_1}(t), & 0 \leq t < t_1, \\ \rho(x_1, x_2)\lambda_{x_1}(t), & t \geq t_1. \end{cases}$$

By the same manner,

$$\begin{aligned} S_{x(\cdot)}(t) &= \begin{cases} S_{x_1}(t), & 0 \leq t < t_1, \\ S_{x_1}(t_1)\frac{S_{x_2}(t)}{S_{x_2}(t_1)}, & t \geq t_1. \end{cases} \\ &= \begin{cases} S_0^{r(x_1)}(t), & 0 \leq t < t_1, \\ S_0^{r(x_1)}(t_1)\left(\frac{S_0(t)}{S_0(t_1)}\right)^{r(x_2)}, & t \geq t_1. \end{cases} \end{aligned}$$

And, for any $x_0 \in E_1$,

$$S_{x(\cdot)}(t) = \begin{cases} S_{x_0}^{\rho(x_0, x_1)}(t), & 0 \leq t < t_1, \\ S_{x_0}^{\rho(x_0, x_1)}(t_1)\left(\frac{S_{x_0}(t)}{S_{x_0}(t_1)}\right)^{\rho(x_0, x_2)}, & t \geq t_1. \end{cases}$$

Taking $x_0 = x_1$ we then obtain

$$S_{x(\cdot)}(t) = \begin{cases} S_{x_1}(t), & 0 \leq t < t_1, \\ S_{x_1}(t_1)\left(\frac{S_{x_1}(t)}{S_{x_1}(t_1)}\right)^{\rho(x_1, x_2)}, & t \geq t_1. \end{cases}$$

The Cox model on E_2 for simple step-stresses of the form (3.3) is known as the *tampered failure rate* (TFR) model (Bhattacharyya and Stoejoeti 1989); see also Bagdonavicius et al. (2002).

3.1.2 Model GM

Let us consider the so-called model GM (*Generalized Multiplicative*) proposed by Bagdonavicius and Nikulin (1995), which generalizes a little the PH model on E. We suppose that there exist a positive function r on E and a survival function S_0 such that for all $x(\cdot) \in E$

$$\frac{\partial f_{x(\cdot)}^G(t)}{\partial t} = r[x(t)]\frac{\partial f_0^G(t)}{\partial t}$$

with the initial conditions

$$f_{x(\cdot)}^G(0) = f_0^G(0) = 0, \quad \text{where} \quad f_0^G(t) = H(S_0(t)), \quad x(\cdot) \in E.$$

We call S_0 the *baseline* survival function. The GM model means that the rate of resource using at the moment t is proportional to some *baseline rate*. The proportionality constant is a function of the stress applied at t.

Taking any two stresses $x(\cdot)$ and $y(\cdot)$ from E we obtain from the definition of the Model GM

$$\frac{\partial f^G_{x(\cdot)}(t)}{\partial t}\Big/\frac{\partial f^G_{y(\cdot)}(t)}{\partial t} = r[x(t)]/r[y(t)],$$

in which one can see that the ratio of resources using at the moment t depends only on the stresses $x(t)$ and $y(t)$. The definition of the model GM implies

$$S_{x(\cdot)}(t) = G\left(\int_0^t r[x(\tau)]dH(S_0(\tau))\right), \quad x(\cdot) \in E.$$

where $H = G^{-1}$. Note that if $x(t) \equiv x = const$, the GM model implies

$$S_{x(\cdot)}(t) = G(r(x)H(S_0(t))), \quad x \in E_1.$$

Consider some *submodels* of GM with G specified. If the distribution of the resource R^G is exponential,

$$G(t) = e^{-t}, \quad t \geq 0,$$

then under the exponential resource we have

$$H = G^{-1}, \quad H(p) = -ln(p), \quad 0 < p < 1,$$

and

$$H(S_0(t)) = -ln S_0(t) = \Lambda_0(t),$$

$$f^G_{x(\cdot)}(t) = H(S_{x(\cdot)}(t)) = -ln S_{x(\cdot)}(t) = \Lambda_{x(\cdot)}(t) = \int_0^t r(x(s))d\Lambda_0(s), \quad x(\cdot) \in E.$$

In this case we obtain the Cox model since

$$\frac{\partial f^G_{x(\cdot)}(t)}{\partial t} = \lambda_{x(\cdot)}(t), \quad x(\cdot) \in E,$$

i.e., the rate of resource using is the hazards rate, and in this case the GM model can be presented by the next way:

$$\lambda_{x(\cdot)}(t) = r(x(t))\lambda_0(t), \quad x(\cdot) \in E.$$

It is the PH model of Cox on E, given by (3.1).

If the distribution of the resource is *log-logistic*,

$$G(t) = \frac{1}{1+t}, \quad t \geq 0,$$

then the GM model can be formulated as

$$\frac{\lambda_{x(\cdot)}(t)}{S_{x(\cdot)}(t)} = r(x(t))\frac{\lambda_0(t)}{S_0(t)}, \quad x(\cdot) \in E.$$

If the stresses are constant in time then we obtain a simple expression on E_1:

$$\frac{1}{S_x(t)} - 1 = r(x)\left(\frac{1}{S_0(t)} - 1\right), \quad x \in E_1.$$

It is the analogue of *logistic regression* model used for the analysis of *dichotomous outcomes* when the probability of *success* depends on some factors. The model given here is close to the Cox model when t is small. It could be useful in practice when the constructed Cox model is not in accordance with the data for small t.

We consider the case when the resource is *lognormal*,

$$G(t) = \Phi(\ln t), \quad t \geq 0,$$

where Φ is the distribution function of the *standard normal law*. If covariates are constant in time then in terms of survival functions the model GM can be written as

$$\Phi^{-1}(S_x(t)) = \ln r(x) + \Phi^{-1}(S_0(t)), \quad x \in E_1.$$

It is the famous *generalized probit model*, see Dabrowska and Doksum (1988).

3.2 Some Simple Examples of Alternatives for the PH Models

Although the PH model works well in many studies, there exist situations when the proportional hazards assumption is not feasible; in particular, when the hazards ratio under different fixed covariates is not constant in time (say, monotone), or when the survivor functions under different stresses intersect, etc. Here are some simple models that could be considered as applicable alternatives to the Cox PH model.

Example 1. Additive Hazard models

The *additive hazard* (AH) model holds on E if the hazard rate under a covariate $x(\cdot)$ is given by

$$\lambda_{x(\cdot)}(t) = \lambda_0(t) + a(x(t)), \quad x(\cdot) \in E.$$

This model is *nonparametric* if $\lambda_0(\cdot)$ and $a(\cdot)$ are unknown functions. The AH model also has the *absence of memory property* as the Cox model, since the value $\lambda_{x(\cdot)}(t)$ of the hazard rate function $\lambda_{x(\cdot)}(\cdot)$ at the moment t does not depend on the values $x(s)$ for $0 < s < t$. That is, the value of the hazard rate function $\lambda_{x(\cdot)}(\cdot)$ does not depend on the history.

The AH model looks very simple on E_1:

$$\lambda_x(t) = \lambda_0(t) + a(x), \quad x \in E_1.$$

The differences of hazard rates for different covariates $x, y \in E_1$ *does not depend* on the baseline function $\lambda_0(\cdot)$ and t:

$$\lambda_x(t) - \lambda_y(t) = a(x) - a(y), \quad x, y \in E_1.$$

The function $a(\cdot)$ is often parameterized as

$$a(x) = \beta^T x, \quad \beta = (\beta_1, \dots, \beta_m)^T.$$

In this case we have the classical *semiparametric* AH regression model on E:

$$\lambda_{x(\cdot)}(t) = \lambda_0(t) + \beta^T x(t), \quad x(\cdot) \in E,$$

which is also known as the *McKeague–Sasieni model* (1994). Application of this model is still restrictive because it does not take into account the history represented by the covariate $x(\cdot)$. For semiparametric analysis of McKeague–Sasieni model, one can refer to Lin and Ying (1994) and Martinussen and Scheike (2006).

Example 2. Model of Lin and Ying

The PH and AH models are special cases of the so-called *additive–multiplicative hazard* (AMH) model on E (Lin and Ying 1996):

$$\lambda_{x(\cdot)}(t) = \beta^T x(t) \lambda_0(t) + \gamma^T x(t), \quad x(\cdot) \in E,$$

where $\gamma = (\gamma_1, \dots, \gamma_m)^T$. Hereafter, it is called the Lin–Ying model. From this formula one can see that Lin–Ying model also has the property of absence of memory.

Example 3. Aalen's additive risk (AAR) model

A different version of the AH model on E_1 was proposed earlier by Aalen (1980). According to the *Aalen's model* on E_1

$$\lambda_x(t) = x^T \lambda_0(t), \quad x \in E,$$

where $\lambda_0(t) = (\lambda_{01}(t), \ldots, \lambda_{0m}(t))^T$ is an unknown vector baseline hazard function, which permits the effects (contribution) of each covariate x_i to be functions of time. Combining the two models (Lin–Ying and AAR) give the well-known *partly parametric additive risk* (PPAR) *model of McKeague and Sasieni* (1994):

$$\lambda_x(t) = y^T \lambda_0(t) + \beta^T z, \quad x(\cdot) \in E_1,$$

where

$$\lambda_0(t) = (\lambda_{01}(t), \ldots, \lambda_{0p}(t))^T, \quad \beta = (\beta_1, \ldots, \beta_q)^T,$$

and

$$y = (x_{1_1}, \ldots x_{1_p})^T \quad \text{and} \quad z = (x_{2_1}, \ldots, x_{2_q})^T$$

are p and q dimensional subvectors ($p \leq m$, $q \leq m$) of the covariate $x = (x_1, \ldots, x_m)^T$.

In general all models considered here are semiparametric, but one can easily parameterize these models as what could be done on the PH model.

3.3 Partial Likelihood Estimation

Consider the set of right-censored data:

$$T_i = \min(T_i^*, C_i), \cdot \text{ and } \delta_i = 1_{\{T_i^* \leq C_i\}}$$

where T_i^* and C_i are survival and censoring times, respectively, associated with the ith individual, and $X_i(t)$ is the time-dependent covariate vector. Let t_i be the realization of T_i. Without loss of generality, we assume $t_1 < \cdots < t_n$ when there are no ties. The partial likelihood proposed by Cox (1972, 1975) is

$$L_p = \prod_i \left\{ \frac{e^{\beta^T X_i(t_i)}}{\sum_j Y_j(t_i) e^{\beta^T X_j(t_i)}} \right\}^{\delta_i}. \tag{3.4}$$

Taking partial derivative of $\log\{L_p\}$ with respect to β, we have the following score function:

$$U(\beta) = \sum_i \left\{ X_i(t_i) - \frac{\sum_j Y_j(t_i) X_j(t_i) e^{\beta^T X_j(t_i)}}{\sum_j Y_j(t_i) e^{\beta^T X_j(t_i)}} \right\}^{\delta_i}. \tag{3.5}$$

Note that, in (3.5), β, $U(\beta)$, and $X(\cdot)$ are all p-dimensional vectors. Setting $U(\beta) = 0$ and using iterative scheme for numerical calculation, we can solve $\widehat{\beta}$ such that $U(\widehat{\beta}) = 0$. For a column vector u, $u^{\otimes 2} = u \cdot u^T$. Further define

$$S^{(0)}(\beta, t) = \frac{1}{n} \sum_i Y_i(t) \exp(\beta^T X_i(t)) \tag{3.6}$$

$$S^{(1)}(\beta, t) = \frac{1}{n} \sum_i Y_i(t) X_i(t) \exp(\beta^T X_i(t)) \tag{3.7}$$

$$S^{(2)}(\beta, t) = \frac{1}{n} \sum_i Y_i(t) X_i(t)^{\otimes 2} \exp(\beta^T X_i(t)) \text{ and} \tag{3.8}$$

$$V(\beta, t) = \frac{S^{(2)}(\beta, t)}{S^{(0)}(\beta, t)} - \left[\frac{S^{(1)}(\beta, t)}{S^{(0)}(\beta, t)} \right]^{\otimes 2}. \tag{3.9}$$

Under suitable regularity conditions (Tsiatis 1981; Andersen et al. 1993), large sample properties of $\widehat{\beta}$ can be obtained. In brief, one can show that $\widehat{\beta}$ is consistent and asymptotic normal:

$$\widehat{\beta} \to_p \beta, \quad \sqrt{n}(\widehat{\beta} - \beta) \to_d N\left(0, \Sigma_\beta^{-1}\right). \tag{3.10}$$

The inverse of the asymptotic variance

$$\Sigma = \int_0^\tau v(\beta, t) s^{(0)}(\beta, t) \lambda_0(t) dt,$$

where the integration is taken over the entire observational time interval $(0, \tau)$, and $v(\beta, t), s^{(0)}(\beta, t), s^{(1)}(\beta, t)$, and $s^{(2)}(\beta, t)$ are the asymptotic limits of

$$V(\beta, t), \ S^{(0)}(\beta, t), \ S^{(1)}(\beta, t) \quad \text{and} \quad S^{(2)}(\beta, t),$$

respectively.

Based on the partial likelihood estimation, the PH analysis has the merits of easy implementation, semiparametric efficient, nice interpretation in hazard ratio, and readily available packages in various statistical softwares (such as SAS, S-plus, R, SPSS, etc.)

3.3.1   Breslow Estimator for the Baseline Cumulative Hazard Function

Once $\widehat{\beta}$ has been obtained, the baseline cumulative hazard can be estimated by

$$\widehat{\Lambda}_0(t) = \sum_{i=1}^n \int_0^t \frac{dN_i(u)}{\sum_j Y_j(t_i) \exp\{\widehat{\beta}^T Z_j(t_i)\}}.$$

It is called the Breslow estimator of $\Lambda_0(t)$ (Breslow 1974). It has been argued that, profiled on $\widehat{\beta}$, the estimator $\widehat{\Lambda}_0(t)$ is the MLE for the full likelihood $L(\beta, \Lambda_0)$; moreover, $L_p(\beta) = \max_{\Lambda_0(\cdot)} L(\beta, \Lambda_0)$ (Johansen 1983; Andersen et al. 1993).

3.3.2 The Stanford Heart Transplant Data as an Example

For the Stanford Heart Transplant (SHT) data introduced in Example 1 of Chap. 1, see Wu and Hsieh (2009) for more explorations. A complete data with 154 observations are used here to implement the conventional PH analysis and compared with the parametric Weibull regression mentioned previously. One can see from the following table that relevant parameter estimates are quite close for the two analysis.

	Cox model	Weibull regression
Variable	Parameter $(\times 10^{-2})$ (p-value)	Parameter $(\times 10^{-2})$ (p-value)
Age	$-12.51(0.0227)$	$-13.34(0.0154)$
Age^2	$0.20(0.0050)$	$0.22(0.0028)$
Mismatch score	$13.71(0.4548)$	$14.79(0.4200)$

The above Weibull regression has the baseline estimate $\widehat{a}t^{\widehat{b}}$, $\widehat{a} = 0.06119$, and $\widehat{b} = 0.5976$. Comparison for the baseline cumulative hazards for the two models (Cox and Weibull) are shown in Fig. 3.1. It exhibits a lower (smaller) estimate for the baseline cumulative hazard using the Cox regression than the parametric Weibull regression.

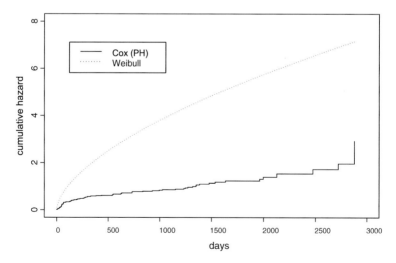

Fig. 3.1 Comparison of baselines: Cox (PH) versus Weibull

3.4   Log-Rank Test and Robust Tests for Treatment Effect

3.4.1   Log-Rank Test and Weighted Log-Rank Test

For the ordered failured times $t_{(1)} < \cdots < t_{(k)}$, let $Z = 1$ codes for the treatment group and $Z = 0$ for the control group. Assume that there are d_i failures observed at $t_{(i)}$, then a 2×2 contingency table is formed as

	Died	Survived	Total
$Z = 1$	d_{1i}	$Y_{1i} - d_{1i}$	Y_{1i}
$Z = 0$	d_{0i}	$Y_{0i} - d_{0i}$	Y_{0i}
total	d_i	$Y_i - d_i$	Y_i

Here Y_{1i} and Y_{0i} are the at-risk number of the group $Z = i$ ($i = 1, 0$) with $Y_i = Y_{1i} + Y_{0i}$, and d_{1i} and d_{0i} are, respectively, the number of failures observed at $t_{(i)}$. Conditional on the marginal totals, the random variable d_{1i} is distributed as a *hypergeometric distribution* with mean and variance:

$$E(d_{1i}) = d_i \frac{Y_{1i}}{Y_i},$$
$$Var(d_{1i}) = d_i \frac{Y_{1i} Y_{0i} (Y_i - d_i)}{Y_i^2 (Y_i - 1)}.$$

By this setting, a series of "correlated" 2×2 tables are formed. However, if the data history satisfies the requirement of *increasing σ-algebras* (a filtration; Sect. 2.3), then the *martingale central limit theorem* can be applied so that

$$\mathscr{T}_{LR} = \frac{\left\{ \sum_{i=1}^k (d_{1i} - E(d_{1i})) \right\}^2}{\sum_{i=1}^k Var(d_{1i})} \tag{3.11}$$

has asymptotically a χ_1^2 distribution. If there are **no ties**, then $d_i = 1$. The log-rank statistic (Mantel 1966; Peto 1972) can be simplified as

$$\mathscr{T}_{LR} = \frac{\left\{ \sum_{i=1}^k (d_{1i} - \bar{d}_{1i}) \right\}^2}{\sum_{i=1}^k \bar{d}_{1i} (1 - \bar{d}_{1i})}, \tag{3.12}$$

where $\bar{d}_{1i} = Y_{1i}/Y_i$ is the sample mean of the indicators of treatment group. A class of *predictable* weight processes $\mathscr{K}(t)$ can be imposed to produce *weighted log-rank* tests (Klein and Moeschberger 1997):

$$\mathscr{T}_{LR} = \frac{\left\{\sum_{i=1}^{k} \mathscr{K}(t_{(i)})(d_{1i} - E(d_{1i}))\right\}^2}{\sum_{i=1}^{k} \mathscr{K}^2(t_{(i)}) Var(d_{1i})}. \tag{3.13}$$

See Sect. 7.3 for more details for the selection of $\mathscr{K}(t)$. It is easy practice to derive the log-rank test as a score test under the proportional hazards model and using the partial likelihood if there are no covariates and the only explanatory variable is the treatment indicator.

3.4.2   Robust Inference: Preliminary

The Cox model (Cox 1972) is the most popular model used in survival analysis for epidemiological data, clinical studies, and many other fields. When there could be model misspecification, robust inferential procedures should be considered. Model misspecification involves several aspects: First, some observations do not actually respond to the covariate in proportional hazards setting. Second, there could be omitted covariates. And, third, variables may have measurement errors. With the general concern of model misspecification, Lin and Wei (1989) derived the asymptotic distribution of the maximum partial likelihood estimator (MPLE) with a *sandwich* variance estimator, and proposed robust tests for treatment effect possibly with covariates adjustment. The procedures suggested in Lin and Wei (1989) are as follows.

Consider a set of random failure times $T_1^*, \ldots, T_n^*$ subject to random right censoring times $C_1, \ldots, C_n$. We observe $T_i = \min(T_i^*, C_i)$ and $\delta_i = 1(T_i^* \leq C_i)$; and $Y_i(t) = 1_{\{T_i \geq t\}}$ is the "at-risk" process. Let the hazard function associated with a set of treatment/covariates be

$$\lambda(t; Z, X) = \lambda_0(t) \exp\{\phi Z + \beta_1 X_1(t) + \cdots + \beta_p X_p(t)\},$$

where Z is the indicator of treatment. Denote $\theta = (\phi, \beta_1, \ldots, \beta_p)^T = (\phi, \beta^T)^T$, $\tilde{X}(t) = (X_1(t), \ldots, X_p(t))^T$, and $X(t) = (Z, \tilde{X}(t)^T)^T$. For individual i, $\lambda_i(t) = \lambda(t; X_i(t))$, $X_i(t) = (Z_i, \tilde{X}_i(t)^T)^T$. Assume that the treatment is assigned by suitable random allocation so that Z is reasonably independent of $\tilde{X}(t)$. Let $l(\theta)$ be the partial likelihood for the "specified" model and further denote

$$H_\theta = -(1/n)\partial^2 l(\theta)/\partial\theta^2 = \begin{pmatrix} H_{\phi\phi} & H_{\phi\beta} \\ H_{\beta\phi} & H_{\beta\beta} \end{pmatrix},$$

$$J_\theta = (1/n)\sum(U_i(\theta)U_i(\theta)^T) = \begin{pmatrix} J_{\phi\phi} & J_{\phi\beta} \\ J_{\beta\phi} & J_{\beta\beta} \end{pmatrix},$$

where $U_i(\theta) = \partial l_i(\theta)/\partial\theta$ with l_i being the contribution from the ith observation to $l(\theta)$; $\sum U_i(\theta) = U_\theta = (U_\phi, U_\beta^T)^T$, $U_\phi = \sum U_{i\phi}$, $U_\beta = \sum U_{i\beta}$.

As was discussed by Lin and Wei (1989) for "fully parametric" problems, a possible *robust* Wald test for $H_0 : \phi = 0$ (means "no treatment effect") is, on one hand,

$$T_{\mathcal{W}1} = n\widehat{\phi}^2\{\widehat{V}_{\phi\phi}\}^{-1},$$

with $\widehat{V}_{\phi\phi}$ being the $(1,1)$th component of $H_\theta^{-1} J_\theta H_\theta^{-1}$ evaluated at $\widehat{\theta} = (0, \widehat{\beta}_0)$, where $\widehat{\beta}_0$ is the restricted MPLE under $H_0 : \phi = 0$. On the other hand, a *robust* score test can be constructed as

$$T_{\mathcal{S}1} = \frac{U_\phi^2(0, \widehat{\beta}_0)}{\sum\{U_{i\phi}(0, \widehat{\beta}_0) - H_{\phi\beta}(0, \widehat{\beta}_0)H_{\beta\beta}^{-1}(0, \widehat{\beta}_0)U_{i\beta}(0, \widehat{\beta}_0)\}^2}.$$

3.4.3 Robust Test with Covariates Adjustment

Lin and Wei's test based on Cox model

We need the following notations:

$$S^{(r)}(t) = n^{-1}\sum_i Y_i(t)\lambda_i(t)X_i(t)^{\otimes r}, \ s^{(r)}(t) = E S^{(r)}(t),$$

$$S^{(r)}(\theta, t) = n^{-1}\sum_i Y_i(t)\exp\{\theta^T X_i(t)\}X_i(t)^{\otimes r}, \ s^{(r)}(\theta, t) = E S^{(r)}(\theta, t),$$

where $r = 0, 1, 2$ and $q^{\otimes 2}$ equals qq^T for a column vector q. With possible model misspecification, assume that there exists a θ^* satisfying

$$\int s^{(1)}(t)dt - \int \frac{s^{(1)}(\theta, t)}{s^{(0)}(\theta, t)}s^{(0)}(t)dt = 0. \tag{3.14}$$

It was proved by Lin and Wei that the MPLE $\widehat{\theta}$ is consistent and asymptotic normal:

$$\sqrt{n}(\widehat{\theta} - \theta^*) \to N(0, H_\theta^{-1} J_\theta^* H_\theta^{-1}),$$

where J_θ^* can be consistently estimated by $\widehat{J}_\theta^*$ calculated at $\widehat{\theta} = (0, \widehat{\beta}_0)$:

$$\widehat{J}_\theta^* = \frac{1}{n}\sum_i \delta_i \left\{\left\{X_i(t) - \frac{S^{(1)}(\theta, t_i)}{S^{(0)}(\theta, t_i)}\right\} - \sum_j \frac{\delta_j Y_i(t_j)e^{\theta^T X_i(t_j)}}{n S^{(0)}(\theta, t_j)}\left\{X_i(t_j) - \frac{S^{(1)}(\theta, t_j)}{S^{(0)}(\theta, t_j)}\right\}\right\}^{\otimes 2}$$

$$\equiv \frac{1}{n}\sum_i \delta_i \mathcal{W}_i^{\otimes 2}, \tag{3.15}$$

The term in the big brackets, $\mathscr{W}_i$, can be decomposed as $(\mathscr{W}_{i\phi}, \mathscr{W}_{i\beta}^T)^T$. Based on this property, Lin and Wei proposed another robust score test:

$$T_{LW} = \frac{U_\phi^2(0, \widehat{\beta}_0)}{\sum\{\mathscr{W}_{i\phi}(0, \widehat{\beta}_0) - H_{\phi\beta}(0, \widehat{\beta}_0)H_{\beta\beta}^{-1}(0, \widehat{\beta}_0)\mathscr{W}_{i\beta}(0, \widehat{\beta}_0)\}^2}. \tag{3.16}$$

The condition (3.14) can be easily interpreted as follows. For individual i, let the hazard of the *true model* be $\lambda_i(t)$ and

$$\lambda(t; Z_i, X_i(t)) = \lambda_0(t)\exp\{\phi Z_i + \beta_1 X_{1i}(t) + \cdots + \beta_p X_{pi}(t)\},$$

be the hazard of the *working model*. For ease of further explorations, assume that under the true model the estimating equation corresponding to the treatment Z can be expressed as

$$\sum \delta_i \left\{ Z_i - \frac{\sum_j Y_j(t_i)\lambda_j(t_i)Z_j}{\sum_j Y_j(t_i)\lambda_j(t_i)} \right\} = 0. \tag{3.17}$$

For the working model, the estimating equation is

$$\sum \delta_i \left\{ Z_i - \frac{\sum_j Y_j(t_i)\exp(\theta^T X_j(t_i))Z_j}{\sum_j Y_j(t_i)\exp(\theta^T X_j(t_i))} \right\} = 0. \tag{3.18}$$

Combining (3.17) and (3.18), we have

$$\frac{1}{n}\sum \delta_i \frac{\frac{1}{n}\sum_j Y_j(t_i)\lambda_j(t_i)Z_j}{\frac{1}{n}\sum_j Y_j(t_i)\lambda_j(t_i)} = \frac{1}{n}\sum \delta_i \frac{\frac{1}{n}\sum_j Y_j(t_i)\exp(\theta^T X_j(t_i))Z_j}{\frac{1}{n}\sum_j Y_j(t_i)\exp(\theta^T X_j(t_i))}. \tag{3.19}$$

According to the arguments of Tsiatis (1981), the left-hand side of (3.19) converges in probability to

$$\int E\left(\frac{1}{n}\sum_j Y_j(t)\lambda_j(t)Z_j\right) dt;$$

and the right-hand side converges to

$$\int \frac{E\left[\frac{1}{n}\sum_j Y_j(t)Z_j\exp\{\theta^T X_j(t)\}\right]}{E\left[\frac{1}{n}\sum_j Y_j(t)\exp\{\theta^T X_j(t)\}\right]} E\left(\frac{1}{n}\sum_j Y_j(t)\lambda_j(t)\right) dt.$$

Or, using the notations in Lin and Wei's paper (1989, formula (2.1)), (3.19) implies

$$\int s^{(1)}(t)dt = \int \frac{s^{(1)}(\theta,t)}{s^{(0)}(\theta,t)} s^{(0)}(t)dt,$$

which is exactly (3.14).

An Improvement
Evidently, Lin and Wei's robust variance estimate $\widehat{H}_\theta^{-1}\widehat{J}_\theta^*\widehat{H}_\theta^{-1}$ can be reexpressed as

$$\frac{1}{n}\sum_i \widehat{IF}_i\widehat{IF}_i^T,$$

where $IF_i = H_\theta^{-1}\mathcal{W}_i$ is the *influence function* and $\widehat{IF}_i$ is the counterpart when the involved θ is replaced by its consistent estimate (Reid and Crépeau 1985; Heritier et al. 2009.) For the purpose of robust estimation, Bednarski (1993) and Minder and Bednarski (1996) proposed an alternative robust procedure based on the following weighted partial score:

$$U_W(\beta) = \sum_i W(t_i, X_i(t_i)) \left\{ X_i(t_i) - \frac{\sum_j Y_j(t_i)W(t_i, X_j(t_i))X_j(t_i)e^{\beta^T X_j(t_i)}}{\sum_j Y_j(t_i)W(t_i, X_j(t_i))e^{\beta^T X_j(t_i)}} \right\}^{\delta_i}.$$

The weight functions appeared at two places have different purposes: for that at the outer sum, it downweights observations with large $t\exp(\beta^T X)$; for the two weights at the numerator and denominator in the curly brackets, they downweight observations with large $\beta^T X$ (Minder and Bednarski 1996). Three basic weights can be used: linear, exponential, and quadratic. We denote the resultant robust estimate as $\widehat{\beta}_{RE}$. Let $\beta = (\phi, \gamma)$ and if the effects of a subset of the covariates are tested, say, $H_0 : \phi = 0$. Then, using the approach of Bednarski (1993) and Minder and Bednarski (1996), robust Wald test and score test can be constructed from replacing the partial score involved in the Lin and Wei's procedure by its counterpart $U_W(\beta)$ and the consistent estimate $\widehat{\beta}_{RE}$. For more details, see Sect. 7.3 of Heritier et al. (2009).

Kong and Slud's Test
Assuming independence between Z and the covariates $\tilde{X}(t)$, Kong and Slud (1997) showed that $U_\phi(0, \widehat{\beta}_0)$ is asymptotically distributed as a zero-mean Gaussian distribution with covariance Σ which can be consistently estimated by

$$\widehat{\Sigma} = \frac{1}{n}\sum_i \delta_i(\mathcal{W}_i^0 - \bar{\mathcal{W}}^0)^2.$$

In the above expression

$$
\mathscr{W}_i^0 = \left\{ Z_i - \frac{\sum_k Z_k Y_k(t_i)}{\sum_k Y_k(t_i)} \right\} - \sum_j \frac{\delta_j Y_i(t_j) e^{\theta^T X_i(t_j)}}{n S^{(0)}(\theta, t_j)} \left\{ Z_i - \frac{\sum_k Z_k Y_k(t_j)}{\sum_k Y_k(t_j))} \right\}
$$

calculated at $\widehat{\theta} = (0, \widehat{\beta}_0)$, and $\bar{\mathscr{W}}^0$ is the sample mean of $\mathscr{W}_i^0 (i = 1, \ldots, n)$. A χ^2-statistic can then be constructed as

$$
T_{KS} = \frac{U_\phi^2(0, \widehat{\beta}_0)}{\frac{1}{n} \sum_i \delta_i \left(\mathscr{W}_i^0 - \bar{\mathscr{W}}^0 \right)^2}. \tag{3.20}
$$

Chapter 4
The AFT, GPH, LT, Frailty, and GLPH Models

4.1 AFT Model

Under the covariate $x(\cdot)$ the probability $S_{x(\cdot)}(t)$ characterizes for any fixed t the summing effect of covariate values in the interval $[0, t]$ on survival. The equality $\Lambda_{x(\cdot)}(t) = -\ln S_{x(\cdot)}(t)$ implies that the cumulative hazard also characterizes this summing effect. So it can be supposed that the hazard rate at any moment t is a function of the covariate value $x(t)$ and the value of the cumulative hazard $\Lambda_{x(\cdot)}(t)$.

The *generalized Sedyakin's* (GS) model on E assumed (Sedyakin 1966)

$$\lambda_{x(\cdot)}(t) = g\left(x(t), \Lambda_{x(\cdot)}(t)\right), \quad x(\cdot) \in E \tag{4.1}$$

with g completely unknown. This model is too general to do statistical inference. However, if we use some regression setting with constant covariates, the form of the function g can be made more concrete.

Let E_1 be a set of constant stresses and E_2 be a set of simple step-stresses of the form

$$x(t) = \begin{cases} x_1, & \text{if } t \le t_1 \\ x_2, & \text{if } t > t_1, \end{cases},$$

where $x_1, x_2 \in E_1$. It is interesting to note that in the GS model the survival function under the simple step-stress is obtained from the survival functions under the constant stresses by the *rule of time-shift*.

One can easily show that, if the GS model holds on E_2, then the survival function and the hazard rate under the stress $x(\cdot) \in E_2$ satisfy the equations

$$S_{x(\cdot)}(t) = \begin{cases} S_{x_1}(t), & \text{if } 0 \le t < t_1, \\ S_{x_2}(t - t_1 + t_1^*), & \text{if } t \ge t_1, \end{cases},$$

and

$$\lambda_{x(\cdot)}(t) = \begin{cases} \lambda_{x_1}(t), & \text{if } 0 \le t < t_1, \\ \lambda_{x_2}(t - t_1 + t_1^*), & \text{if } t \ge t_1, \end{cases}$$

© The Author(s) 2016
M. Nikulin and H.-D.I. Wu, *The Cox Model and Its Applications*,
SpringerBriefs in Statistics, DOI 10.1007/978-3-662-49332-8_4

respectively, where the moment t_1^* is determined by the next equation

$$S_{x_1}(t_1) = S_{x_2}(t_1^*).$$

From these equations we obtain the Sedyakin's model according to which

$$\lambda_{x(\cdot)}(t_1 + s) = \lambda_{x_2}(t_1^* + s), \quad s \geq 0.$$

Suppose that under different constant covariates $x \in E_1$ the survival functions differ only in scale:

$$S_x(t) = S_0(r(x)t), \quad x \in E_1, \tag{4.2}$$

for some positive r on E_1. If the GS model holds on a set E, $E \supset E_1$, of covariates, then (2) holds on E_1 if and only if the function g has the form $g(x, s) = r(x)q(s)$ for some positive q (Fig. 4.1).

So, we obtain the following model:

$$\lambda_{x(\cdot)}(t) = r\{x(t)\}\, q\{\Lambda_{x(\cdot)}(t)\}, \quad x(\cdot) \in E. \tag{4.3}$$

Using the relation between the survival and the cumulative hazard functions, it is easy to obtain the so-called AFT (*accelerated failure time*) model on E according to which the survival function has the form

$$S_{x(\cdot)}(t) = S_0\left(\int_0^t r(x(u))du\right), \quad x(\cdot) \in E, \tag{4.4}$$

Fig. 4.1 Cumulative distribution function under Sedykin's principle for increasing step-stress from $\in E_2$

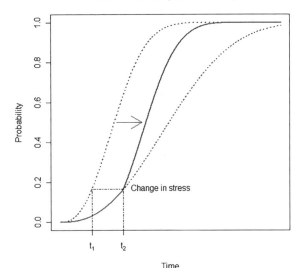

where the function S_0 does not depend on $x(\cdot)$. The function r changes locally with time, and is often parameterized as:

$$r(x) = e^{-\beta^T x},$$

where $\beta = (\beta_1, \ldots, \beta_m)^T$ is a vector of unknown regression parameters.

Under the parameterized AFT model the survival function is

$$S_{x(\cdot)}(t) = S_0 \left(\int_0^t e^{-\beta^T x(u)} du \right), \quad x(\cdot) \in E, \tag{4.5}$$

and the hazard rate is

$$\lambda_{x(\cdot)}(t) = e^{-\beta^T x(t)} \lambda_0 \left(\int_0^t e^{-\beta^T x(u)} du \right), \quad x(\cdot) \in E \tag{4.6}$$

For constant covariates,

$$S_x(t) = S_0 \left(e^{-\beta^T x} t \right), \quad x \in E_1.$$

The AFT model on E_1 can also be written as a *log-linear* model or *linear transformation* (LT) model, since the logarithm of the failure time T_x under constant covariate x can be written as

$$\ln\{T_x\} = \beta^T x + \varepsilon, \quad x \in E_1, \tag{4.7}$$

where the survival function of the random variable ε does not depend on x and $S(t) = S_0(\ln t)$.

In the case of lognormal, the distribution of ε is normal and we have the standard linear regression model. The equality (4.6) implies that if the survival function under any constant covariate belongs to parametric families such as Weibull, log-logistic, and lognormal, then the survival function under any other constant covariate also belongs to that family. The survival functions under any $x_1, x_2 \in E_1$ are related in the following way:

$$S_{x_2}(t) = S_{x_1}\{\rho(x_1, x_2)t\}, \quad t > 0,$$

where

$$\rho(x_1, x_2) = \frac{r(x_2)}{r(x_1)}.$$

Using the relations between the GS and AFT models we can find the form of the survival functions for AFT model under simple step-stresses. Indeed, if the AFT model holds on E_2 then the survival function under any stress $x(\cdot) \in E_2$ of the form (3.3) satisfies the equality

$$S_{x(\cdot)}(t) = \begin{cases} S_{x_1}(t), & \text{if } 0 \le t < t_1, \\ S_{x_2}(t - t_1 + t_1^*), & \text{if } t \ge t_1, \end{cases}$$

where

$$t_1^* = \frac{r(x_1)}{r(x_2)}t.$$

Different from the PH model, the AFT model is mostly applied in survival analysis as a parametric model: the function S_0 (or the distribution of ε) is taken from some parametric class of distributions.

In the case of semiparametric estimation the function S_0 is assumed to be completely unknown and in model (4.5) the regression parameters as well as the function S_0 needs to be estimated. The semiparametric AFT model is much less used in survival analysis than the Cox's PH model because of complicated estimation procedures: modified variants of likelihood functions are not differentiable and even not continuous functions; the limit covariance matrices of the regression parameters depend on the derivatives of the probability density functions.

The parametric AFT model is used in failure time regression analysis and accelerated life testing. Under special experiment plans even nonparametric estimation procedures are used. In such a case not only the function S_0 but also the function r in the model (4.4) is assumed to be completely unknown.

The AFT model is a good choice when the lifetime distribution class is supposed to be known. Nevertheless, it is as restrictive as the PH model. The assumption that the survival distributions under different covariate values differ only in scale is a rather strong assumption. So more sophisticated models are also needed. For more properties and different biomedical applications about the AFT model, see Meeker and Escobar (1998), Bagdonavičius and Nikulin (2002b, c), Dabrowska (2005–2006), and Martinussen and Scheike (2006).

Remark 1. The PH and AFT models are equivalent on E_1 if and only if the failure time distribution is Weibull for all $x \in E_1$.

Remark 2. (Changing shape and scale (CHSS) models)
If a natural generalization of the AFT model (4.4) is obtained, different constant stresses x influence both scale and shape of a survival distribution (Mann et al. 1974):

$$S_x(t) = S_0 \left\{ \left(\frac{t}{\sigma(x)} \right)^{\nu(x)} \right\},$$

where σ and ν some positive functions on E_1. Generalization of this model to include time-dependent covariates is the *changing shape and scale* (CHSS) model, (Bagdonavičius et al. 1999, 2004):

$$S_{x(\cdot)}(t) = S_0 \left(\int_0^t r\{x(u)\} u^{\nu(x(u))-1} du \right). \qquad (4.8)$$

In this model the variation of stress changes locally not only the scale but also the shape of distribution.

In terms of the default rate functions the model can be written in the form:

$$\lambda_{x(\cdot)}(t) = r\{x(t)\}\, q(\Lambda_{x(\cdot)}(t))\, t^{\nu(x(t))-1}, \qquad (4.9)$$

where $q(u) = \lambda_0(\Lambda_0^{-1}(u))$, $\Lambda_0(t) = -\ln S_0(t)$, $\lambda_0(t) = \Lambda_0'(t)$. If $\nu(x) \equiv 1$ then the model coincides with the AFT model with $r(x) = 1/\sigma(x)$. The CHSS model is not in the class of the GPH models (Chap. 4) because the third factor at the right of the formula (4.9) depends not only on t but also on $x(t)$.

The CHSS model is parametric, if S_0 is taken from some parametric class of survival functions and the functions r and ν are parameterized; for example, taking $r(x) = e^{\beta^T x}$, $\nu(x) = e^{\gamma x}$. The model is *semiparametric* if the function S_0 is considered as unknown and the functions r and ν are parameterized as:

$$\lambda_{x(\cdot)}(t) = e^{\beta^T x(t)}\, q(\Lambda_{x(\cdot)}(t))\, t^{\exp\{\gamma^T x(t)\}-1}. \qquad (4.10)$$

For various classes of S_0 the CHSS model includes cross-effect of survival functions under constant covariates. For example, if the survival distribution under constant covariates is Weibull or log-logistic, there exists cross-effects.

Parametric analysis can be done by using the method of maximum likelihood. If semiparametric analysis is considered, the estimation procedure is more complicated because the same problems as in the case of AFT semiparametric model arise: modified variants of likelihood functions are not differentiable and even not continuous functions, the limit covariance matrices of the normed regression parameters depend on the derivatives of the probability density functions.

For more about the PH model and its relations with other models, see Bagdonavicius and Nikulin (2002).

4.2 The GPH Models

The AFT and PH models are rather restrictive. Under the PH model, lifetime distributions with constant covariates are from a narrow class of distributions: the *ratio of hazard rates* (or simply *hazard ratio*, abbreviated as "HR") with respect to any two different constant covariates is constant over time. Under the AFT model the covariate changes (locally, if the covariate is not constant) only the scale.

On the other hand, the *generalized proportional hazards* (GPH) model on E, proposed by Bagdonavičius and Nikulin (1995,1997a,b,1999), allows the hazard ratio associated with two constant covariates to be *time-dependent*. They include AFT and PH models as special cases.

The survival function $S_{x(\cdot)}(t)$ (or, equivalently, the cumulative hazard function $\Lambda_{x(\cdot)}(t)$) characterizes the summing effect of covariate values in the interval $[0, t]$ on survival. So it is reasonable to assume that the hazard rate at any moment t is proportional to a function of the covariate applied at this moment, to a baseline rate, and to a function of the probability of survival until t (or, equivalently, to the cumulative hazard at t):

$$\lambda_{x(\cdot)}(t) = r\{x(t)\}\, q\{\Lambda_{x(\cdot)}(t)\}\, \lambda_0(t), \quad x(\cdot) \in E. \tag{4.11}$$

We call model (4.11) the generalized proportional hazards (GPH) model, see Bagdonavičius and Nikulin (1999), Dabrowska (2005–2007), Martinussen and Scheike (2006). The GPH model includes as special examples the PH model ($q(u) \equiv 1$) and the AFT model ($\lambda_0(t) \equiv \lambda_0 = const$).

Under the GPH model on E the survival functions $S_{x(\cdot)}$ have the form

$$S_{x(\cdot)}(t) = G\left\{\int_0^t r(x(\tau))d\Lambda_0(t)\right\}, \quad x(\cdot) \in E, \tag{4.12}$$

where

$$\Lambda_0(t) = \int_0^t \lambda_0(u)du, \quad G = H^{-1}, \quad H(u) = \int_0^{-\ln u} \frac{dv}{q(v)}.$$

We denote by H^{-1} the function inverse to G.

With regard to (4.11), models with different levels of generality can be obtained by completely specifying q, parameterizing q, or considering q as unknown. However, complete specification of q gives rather strict models which are alternatives to the PH model and the field of their application is relatively limited (Bagdonavičius and Nikulin 1994). Under constant covariates such models are the *linear transformation* (LT) models, proposed by Dabrowska and Doksum (1988). Indeed, if q is specified and r is parameterized by $r(x) = e^{\beta^T x}$, then under constant covariables the survival functions have the form

$$S_{x(\cdot)}(t) = G\left\{e^{\beta^T x}\Lambda_0(t)\right\}, \quad x \in E_1,$$

with G specified. This implies that the random variable T_x can be transformed by the function $h(t) = \ln\{H(S_0(t))\}$ to the random variable of the form

$$h(T_x) = -\beta^T x + \varepsilon, \quad x \in E_1 \tag{4.13}$$

where ε is a random error with the parameter-free distribution function

$$Q(u) = 1 - G(e^u).$$

It is the LT model of Dabrowska and Doksum (1988), Dabrowska (2005–2007).

Examples of the LT models include:

(1) PH model (G is the Weibull survival function, ε has the extreme value distribution).
(2) Proportional odds model (G is the log-logistic survival function, ε has the logistic distribution):

$$\frac{1}{S_x(t)} - 1 = r(x)\left(\frac{1}{S_0(t)} - 1\right), \quad x \in E_1,$$

see Bennett (1983), Murphy et al. (1997), Yang and Prentice (1999). For more about semiparametric estimation for LT models, see Dabrowska (2005–2007), Martinussen and Scheke (2006), Chen et al. (2002), and Bagdonavičius and Nikulin (1999).
(3) Generalized probit model (G is a lognormal and ε has a normal distribution):

$$\Phi^{-1}(S_x(t)) = \log(r(x)) + \Phi^{-1}(S_0(t)), \quad x \in E_1,$$

where Φ is the standard normal cumulative distribution function.

The last two models are alternatives to the PH model. They are widely used for analysis of dichotomous data when the probability of "success" depending on some factors is analyzed. If application of the PH model is dubious then it is better to use a wider GPH model by taking a simple parametric model for the function q.

Let us consider the relationship between the GPH models and the *frailty models* (Hougaard 2000) with covariates. For the frailty model, the hazard rate is influenced not only by the observable covariate $x(\cdot)$ but also by a non-observable positive random covariate Z, called the *frailty variable*. Suppose that, given the frailty variable, the hazard rate is

$$\lambda_{x(\cdot)}(t|Z=z) = z\,r(x(t))\,\lambda_0(t), \quad x(\cdot) \in E.$$

Then

$$S_{x(\cdot)}(t) = \mathbf{E}\,exp\{-Z\int_0^t r(x(\tau))\,d\Lambda_0(\tau)\} = G\{\int_0^t r(x(\tau))d\Lambda_0(\tau)\},$$

where $G(s) = \mathbf{E}e^{-sZ}$. So the GPH model can be defined by suitably specifying the distribution of the frailty variable.

4.3 The GPH Models with Monotone Hazard Ratios

The following parameterizations of r and q give submodels of the GPH model with monotone hazard ratio under constant covariates. Using only one parameter and power (or exponential) function for the parameterization of q, several important models were obtained by Bagdonazvicius and Nikulin (1999).

Suppose that $q(0) = 1$ (if it is not so, we can include $q(0)$ in λ_0, which is considered as unknown), and taking a power function $q(u) = (1 + u)^{-\gamma+1}$ and $r(x) = e^{\beta^T x}$, we obtain the first GPH model (GPH1) on E:

$$\lambda_{x(\cdot)}(t) = e^{\beta^T x(t)}\{1 + \Lambda_{x(\cdot)}(t)\}^{-\gamma+1}\lambda_0(t), \quad x(\cdot) \in E. \tag{4.14}$$

It coincides with the PH model when $\gamma = 1$. The support of the survival function $S_{x(\cdot)}$ is $[0, \infty)$ when $\gamma \geq 0$ and $[0, sp_{x(\cdot)})$ with finite right ends $sp_{x(\cdot)}$, $sp_{x(\cdot)} < \infty$, when $\gamma < 0$. Finite supports are very possible in accelerated life testing: failures of units at different accelerated stresses are concentrated in intervals with different finite right limits.

Suppose that at the point $t = 0$ the hazard ratio $HR(t, x_1, x_2)$ under constant covariates x_1 and x_2 is greater then 1:

$$HR(0, x_1, x_2) = \frac{r(x_2)}{r(x_1)} = c_0 > 1, \quad x_1, x_2 \in E_1,$$

then the hazard ratio $HR(t, x_1, x_2)$ has the following properties:

(a) if $\gamma > 1$, HR decreases from $c_0 > 1$ to $c_\infty = c_0^{\frac{1}{\gamma}} \in (1, c_0)$;
(b) if $\gamma = 1$ (PH model), HR is constant;

(c) if $0 \leq \gamma < 1$, then HR increases from c_0 to $c_\infty = c_0^{\frac{1}{\gamma}} \in (c_0, \infty)$.
(d) if $\gamma < 0$, HR increases from c_0 to ∞ and the infinity is attained at

$$sp_{x_2} = \Lambda_0^{-1}\{-1/(r(x_2) \cdot \gamma)\}.$$

The hazard rates go away from each other quickly when t increases.

The GPH1 model is a generalization of the *positive stable frailty model*. The GPH model with $\gamma = 1/\alpha > 0$ is obtained by taking the frailty variable Z which follows the positive stable distribution with the density

$$p_Z(z) = -\frac{1}{\pi z}\exp\{-\alpha z + 1\}\sum_{k=1}^{\infty}\frac{(-1)^k}{k!}\sin(\pi\alpha k)\frac{\Gamma(\alpha k + 1)}{z^{\alpha k}}, \quad z > 0,$$

where α is a stable index, $0 < \alpha < 1$. For more details, see Bagdonavicius and Nikulin (2002), Greenwood and Nikulin (1996).

4.4   The Second GPH Model

Under the GPH1 model the support of the survival function is infinite when $\gamma \geq 0$ and finite when $\gamma < 0$. The limit is $\gamma = 1$. Taking the parameterization $q(u) = (1 + \gamma u)^{-1}$, we obtain the second GPH (GPH2) model on E:

$$\lambda_{x(\cdot)}(t) = e^{\beta^T x(t)}(1 + \gamma \Lambda_{x(\cdot)}(t))^{-1}\lambda_0(t), \quad \gamma \geq 0, \quad x(\cdot) \in E. \tag{4.15}$$

It also coincides with the PH model when $\gamma = 0$. The supports of the survival functions $S_{x(\cdot)}$ are $[0, \infty)$.

The hazard ratio

$$HR(t, x_1, x_2) = \lambda_{x_2}(t)/\lambda_{x_1}(t), \quad x_1, x_2 \in E_1,$$

has the following properties:

(a) if $\gamma > 0$, then HR decreases from $c_0 > 1$ to the value $\sqrt{c_0} \in (1, c_0)$, i.e., the hazard rates approach each other when t increases;
(b) if $\gamma = 0$ (PH model), the HR is constant.

The GPH2 model is equivalent to the *inverse Gaussian frailty model*. The GPH model with $\gamma = (4\sigma\theta)^{1/2} > 0$ is obtained from taking Z, the frailty variable, to follow the inverse Gaussian distribution with the density

$$p_Z(z) = \left(\frac{\sigma}{\pi}\right)^{1/2} e^{\sqrt{4\sigma\theta}} z^{-3/2} e^{-\theta z - \sigma/z}, \quad z > 0.$$

See Voinov and Nikulin (1993, 1996) for more details.

4.5 The GLPH Model

Taking the exponential functions $q(u) = e^{-\gamma u}$ and $r(x) = e^{\beta^T x}$ we have the third GPH (GPH3) model:

$$\lambda_{x(\cdot)}(t) = e^{\beta^T x(t) - \gamma \Lambda_{x(\cdot)}(t)} \lambda_0(t), \quad x(\cdot) \in E. \tag{4.16}$$

This model is also known as the GLPH (generalized linear PH) model which coincides with the PH model when $\gamma = 0$; (see Bagdonavicus et al. 2000, 2002). The support of the survival function $S_{x(\cdot)}$ is $[0, \infty)$ when $\gamma \geq 0$, or is $[0, sp_{x(\cdot)})$ with finite right ends when $\gamma < 0$.

Suppose that $HR(0, x_1, x_2) = r(x_2)/r(x_1) = c_0 > 1$. The hazard ratio $HR(t, x_1, x_2), x_1, x_2 \in E_1$, has the following properties:

(a) if $\gamma > 0$, then HR decreases from the value $c > 0$ to 1; i.e., the hazard rates approach each other and meet at infinity;
(b) if $\gamma = 0$ (PH model), the HR is constant;
(c) if $\gamma < 0$, HR increases from $c_0 > 1$ to ∞, and the infinity is attained at $sp_{x_2} = \Lambda_0^{-1}\{-1/(\gamma r(x_2))\}$. The hazard rates go away from each other quickly when t increases.

The GPH3 model is a generalization of the *gamma frailty model with explanatory variables*: the GPH model with $\gamma = 1/k > 0$ is obtained taking the frailty variable Z which follows the gamma distribution with the density

$$p_Z(z) = \frac{z^{k-1}}{\theta^k \Gamma(k)} e^{-z/\theta}, \quad z > 0.$$

All the three GPH models are considered as semiparametric; β, γ, and the baseline function Λ_0 are unknown parameters.

Chapter 5
Cross-Effect Models of Survival Functions

In this chapter and Chap. 6, we introduce several models which can deal with cross-effect; including the Hsieh model and the simple cross-effect (SCE) model. Cross-effect is a common phenomenon that appeared in survival data collected from clinical trials, epidemiologic studies, and medical fields. A famous example is the data of the Gastrointestinal Tumor Study Group concerning the effect of chemotherapy versus radiotherapy on the survival times of gastric cancer patients (Stablein and Koutrou-velis 1985; see Chap. 1). To deal with the cross effect, Hsieh (2001) considered a quite general non-proportional hazards model and suggested the over identified estimating equation (OEE) approach with sieve approximation to the baseline hazard. (See Sect. 5.4 for more details.)

In contrast to the Hsieh model, a simple cross-effect (SCE) model was proposed in Bagdonavičius, Hafdi and Nikulin (2004), Bagdonavičius, Levuliene, Nikulin and Cheminade (2004), Bagdonavičius and Nikulin (2005). It has the advantage that the hazard ratio is finite under different covariates at time zero. A natural generalization of the Nelson–Aalen estimator of the baseline function is considered and efficient semiparametric estimation based on the likelihood function is proposed. These two models (Hsieh and SCE) are flexible in that they accommodate mixed type regressors: dichotomous, polytomous, or continuous covariates.

We analyze the gastric cancer data (Fig. 1.3) and compare the estimates of the two survivals based on the Hsieh model and the SCE model in Chap. 6. See also Hsieh (2001), Kleinbaum and Klein (2005), Klein and Moeschberger (2003), and Zeng and Lin (2007). Before the presentation of statistical inferences of the Hsieh and SCE models, we introduce several alternative models which are also capable of capturing cross-effect phenomenon: (a) the change-point model; (b) the parametric *generalized* Weibull regression model which considers modeling the shape-parameter by a regressive component; and (c) the varying-coefficient Cox type regression.

© The Author(s) 2016
M. Nikulin and H.-D.I. Wu, *The Cox Model and Its Applications*,
SpringerBriefs in Statistics, DOI 10.1007/978-3-662-49332-8_5

5.1 Change Point Model

Liang et al. (1990) proposed a change-point model suitable for fitting a Cox-type model with different hazard-ratio parameters for early and late onset of a disease.

$$\lambda(t|X, Z) = \lambda_0(t) \exp\{\beta^T X + (\gamma + \theta 1_{\{t \le \tau\}})Z\}, \tag{5.1}$$

where τ, called the *change point*, is the parameter ranging from a to b (with a and b both known). For the set of ordered *uncensored* times $t_1 < \cdots < t_k$, they proposed to test for the cross-effect $H_0 : \theta = 0$ versus $H_a : \theta \ne 0$ by considering the following (log-) partial likelihood:

$$l = \log\left\{\prod_{i=1}^{k} \frac{\exp\{\beta^T X_i(t_i) + (\gamma + \theta 1_{\{t_i \le \tau\}})Z_i(t_i)\}}{\sum_j Y_j(t_i) \exp\{\beta^T X_j(t_i) + (\gamma + \theta 1_{\{t_i \le \tau\}})Z_j(t_i)\}}\right\}.$$

Let $\phi = (\beta^T, \gamma)^T$ and define

$$S(\tau) = \frac{\partial l}{\partial \theta} \Bigg/ \left\{\frac{-\partial^2 l}{\partial \theta^2} - \left(\frac{-\partial^2 l}{\partial \theta \partial \phi}\right)^T \left(\frac{-\partial^2 l}{\partial \phi^2}\right)^{-1} \left(\frac{-\partial^2 l}{\partial \theta \partial \phi}\right)\right\}^{\frac{1}{2}},$$

which is to be evaluated at $\widehat{\phi} = (\widehat{\beta}^T, \widehat{\gamma})^T$ under $H_0 : \theta = 0$. Then the statistic

$$\mathscr{M} = \sup_{\tau \in [a,b]} S(\tau)$$

can be used to define a *possible* estimate of τ (denoted $\widehat{\tau}$) and the asymptotic distribution of $\mathscr{M}$ is derived as being the supremum of a normalized *Brownian bridge* process. Conditioning on $\widehat{\tau}$, Liang et al. claimed that simultaneous confidence interval construction can be made based on l.

5.2 Parametric Weibull Regression with Heteroscedastic Shape Parameter

As illustrated in the parametric example of Cox model in Chap. 3, if the Weibull class has a shape parameter (b) which can be further modeled as $b = \exp(\gamma^T X)$, then

$$\Lambda(t; X) = \{at^{\exp(\gamma^T X)}\}e^{\beta^T X}$$

or

$$\lambda(t; X) = ae^{(\beta+\gamma)^T X} t^{\exp(\gamma^T X)-1}.$$

For illustrative purpose, consider the simplest case (i.e., two-sample problem) that X is univariate and binary: $X = 0$ or 1. The hazard ratio $(HR(t))$, which is time dependent, between the two groups $\lambda(t; X = 1)$ versus $\lambda(t; X = 0)$ is

$$HR(t) = \phi t^{\sigma - 1}, \text{ where } \sigma = e^{\gamma}, \phi = e^{\beta + \gamma}.$$

The case $\sigma = 1$ or $\gamma = 0$ corresponds to the proportional-hazards setting; and $HR(t)$ is increasing or decreasing for $\sigma > 1$ ($\gamma > 0$) and $\sigma < 1$ ($\gamma < 0$), respectively. The *cross point* of these two hazard functions can be easily solved as

$$t = \exp\left(\frac{\beta + \gamma}{1 - \sigma}\right).$$

In this case, it should be noted that the cross point of the corresponding *cumulative hazards* is $t = \exp\{\beta/(1 - \sigma)\}$.

A question arises when the heteroscedastic Weibull regression is used: At $\sigma < 1$ ($\gamma < 0$), $HR(t) \to \infty$ as $t \to 0$. The following small amendment on the cumulative hazard offers a remedy to the mathematically unpleasant situation:

$$\Lambda(t; X) = a\{(1 + t)^{\exp(\gamma^T X)} - 1\}e^{\beta^T X}.$$

This gives $\Lambda(t; X) = 0$ when $t = 0$ and

$$\lambda(t; X) = ae^{(\beta + \gamma)^T X}(1 + t)^{\exp(\gamma^T X) - 1}.$$

Again, for the two-sample example,

$$HR(t) = \phi(1 + t)^{\sigma - 1}.$$

The pattern of $HR(t)$ and the cross point of the hazard rates remain. However, the cross point of the cumulative hazards satisfies $t = \exp(\beta)\{(1 + t)^{\sigma} - 1\}$.

5.3 Cox-Type Model with Varying Coefficients

The proportional hazards model can be extended to modeling cross-effect by incorporating varying coefficients:

$$\lambda(t; X) = \lambda_0(t) \exp\{\beta(t)^T X(t)\}, \tag{5.2}$$

where $X(t)$ is a p-dimensional time-dependent covariate and $\beta(t)$ is the associated smooth time-varying coefficient. With model (5.2), Murphy and Sen (1991), Murphy (1993), and Marzec and Marzec (1997) considered *sieve approximation* to the varying coefficient(s). Estimation procedures and goodness-of-fit problems were studied in these works.

On the other hand, Cai and Sun (2003) and Tian et al. (2005) (TZW) considered *local smoothing* technique to construct inferential basis. Using the notations and terminology of TZW, for a given time t the *local log partial likelihood* is

$$\mathscr{L}(\beta, t) = \frac{1}{nh_n} \sum_{i=1}^{n} \int_0^{\tau} K\left(\frac{s-t}{h_n}\right) \left\{ \beta^T X_i(s) - \log\left(\sum_j Y_j(s) e^{\beta^T X_j(s)}\right) \right\} dN_i(s),$$
(5.3)

where τ is the prespecified maximal observation time; $K(\cdot)$, the kernel function, is a probability density function symmetric about 0 with mean 0 and *support* $[-1, 1]$. By this, only observations lying in the h_n-neighborhood of t are included; $h_n = O(n^{-\nu})$, $\nu > 0$. The maximizer of $\mathscr{L}$, denoted $\widehat{\beta}(t)$, needs cautious specification close to the time *boundaries* of the study: $\widehat{\beta}(t) = \widehat{\beta}(h_n)$ for $0 < t < h_n$ and $\widehat{\beta}(t) = \widehat{\beta}(\tau - h_n)$ for $\tau - h_n < t < \tau$. In brief, for $t \in [h_n, \tau - h_n]$, the maximizer $\widehat{\beta}(t)$ satisfies $\mathscr{U}(\beta, t) = 0$ where

$$\mathscr{U}(\beta, t) = \frac{1}{\sqrt{n}h_n} \sum_{i=1}^{n} \int_0^{\tau} K\left(\frac{s-t}{h_n}\right) \left\{ X_i(s) - \frac{\sum_j Y_j(s) X_j(s) e^{\beta^T X_j(s)}}{\sum_j Y_j(s) e^{\beta^T X_j(s)}} \right\} dN_i(s).$$
(5.4)

Asymptotic properties of this estimation procedure are studied in Cai and Sun (2003) and Tian et al. (2005). For more theoretical discussions on the estimation and applications, see Martinussen and Scheike (2006).

5.4   Hsieh Model

Hsieh (2001) considers explicit modeling of crossing hazards by including a heteroscedasticity parameter in the power of the baseline cumulative hazard:

$$\Lambda(t; X) = \{\Lambda_0(t)\}^{\sigma} \exp\{\beta^T X\}, \quad \sigma = \exp(\gamma^T X), \tag{5.5}$$

where X is a p-vector and $\Lambda_0(\cdot)$ is an unspecified baseline cumulative hazard. In terms of hazard function, formula (5.5) is expressed as

$$\lambda(t; X) = \lambda_0(t) \exp\{\beta^T X\} \sigma \{\Lambda_0(t)\}^{\sigma-1}. \tag{5.6}$$

In fact, this heteroscedastic model is originally obtained from the linear transformation model with heteroscedastic errors (Hsieh 2001). Different models corresponding to different transforms are listed in Hsieh (1995, p. 741).

The heterogeneity effect can be explored by taking one-dimensional case as an example. The log-hazard ratio ($\equiv$ log HR(t)) between X_1 versus X_0 ($X_1 - X_0 = 1$) is

$$\log\{\mathrm{HR}(t)\} = (e^{\gamma X_1} - e^{\gamma X_0}) \log \Lambda_0(t) + (\beta + \gamma). \tag{5.7}$$

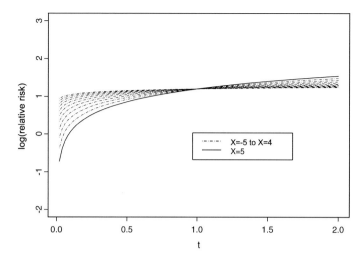

Fig. 5.1 Hsieh model, gamma = 0.2. Reprinted from Statistics and Modelling in Public Health, H.-D.I. Wu, Statistical Inference for Two-Sample and Regression Models with Heterogeneity Effect: A Collected-Sample Perspective, pp. 452–465, Copyright 2006, with permission from Springer

If log HR(t) is of concern, (5.7) implies that the effect is *time-varying*, and it also depends on the value of X. Figures 5.1 and 5.2 illustrate how the log HR depends on t and on X: Let $X_j = -5, -4, \ldots, 5$, and $\gamma = 0.2$ (Fig. 5.1), and 0.5 (Fig. 5.2); $\beta = 1$ for both cases. When the heteroscedasticity parameter is small ($\gamma = 0.2$, Fig. 5.1),

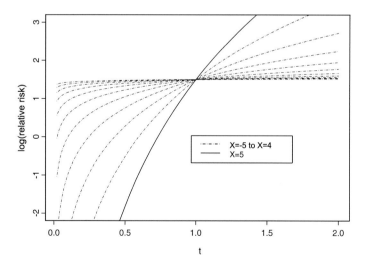

Fig. 5.2 Hsieh model, gamma = 0.5. Reprinted from Statistics and Modelling in Public Health, H.-D.I. Wu, Statistical Inference for Two-Sample and Regression Models with Heterogeneity Effect: A Collected-Sample Perspective, pp. 452–465, Copyright 2006, with permission from Springer

the log HR(t) looks more like a constant in time for some X and they also coincide for much of the time $t \in (0, 2)$. For larger γ, time-dependence of log HR(t) is more obvious. Moreover, for fixed t, log HR(t) differs for different X values, revealing non-ignorable heterogeneity. For both figures, only $X = 5$ is plotted by a solid line to present the trend of log(HR)-plot in X (Wu 2006).

5.4.1   Estimating Equation Processes

Denote the intensity process associated with the ith individual by $\lambda(t; X_i)$, and the counting process recording the observed failure of individual i up to time t by $N_i(t)$. Define

$$S_J(t) = \frac{1}{n} \sum Y_i(t) J_i(t) \exp\{\beta^T X_i\} \sigma_i \{\Lambda_0(t)\}^{\sigma_i - 1}$$

for any predictable $J(t)$; for examples,

$$S_1 = \frac{1}{n} \sum Y_i(t) \exp\{\beta^T X_i\} \sigma_i \{\Lambda_0(t)\}^{\sigma_i - 1}$$

and

$$S_X = \frac{1}{n} \sum Y_i(t) X_i(t) \exp\{\beta^T X_i\} \sigma_i \{\Lambda_0(t)\}^{\sigma_i - 1},$$

etc. Estimating equations for $\Lambda_0(\cdot)$, β and γ are

$$M_1(t) = \Lambda_0(t) - \sum \int_0^t \frac{dN_i(u)}{\sum Y_i(u) \exp\{\beta^T X_i\} \sigma_i \{\Lambda_0(u)\}^{\sigma_i - 1}}, \qquad (5.8)$$

$$M_2(t) = \sum \int_0^t \left\{ X_i - \frac{S_X(u; \Lambda_0, \theta)}{S_1(u; \Lambda_0, \theta)} \right\} dN_i(u), \qquad (5.9)$$

and

$$M_3(t) = \sum \int_0^t \left\{ V_i - \frac{S_V(u; \Lambda_0, \theta)}{S_1(u; \Lambda_0, \theta)} \right\} dN_i(u), \qquad (5.10)$$

where

$$\sigma_i = \exp(\gamma^T X_i) \quad \text{and} \quad V_i(t) = X_i(t) \exp(\gamma^T X_i) \log\{\Lambda_0(t)\}.$$

These estimating equations can be solved with a sieve approximation of the $\Lambda_0(\cdot)$. In fact, the estimating functions (M_2 and M_3) can be derived as follows:

   According to either (5.5) or (5.6), the full likelihood, L_F, with Johansen's decomposition (Johansen 1983) is

$$L_F(\beta, \gamma, \Lambda_0) = \prod \int_0^\tau \frac{h_i(u)dN_i(u)}{\lambda_0(u)S_1(u)} \cdot \prod \int_0^\tau \lambda_0(u)S_1(u)dN_i(u)e^{-\int_0^\tau n\lambda_0(u)S_1(u)du}$$

The first term in the product is the *partial likelihood*. Let

$$l_p = \sum \log \left\{ \int_0^\tau \frac{h_i(u)dN_i(u)}{\lambda_0(u)S_1(u)} \right\}.$$

Taking partial derivatives of l_p with respect to β and γ leads to M_2 and M_3.

5.4.2 Sieve Approximation

Let $\{t_i\}_1^n$ be the realizations of $\{T_i\}_{i=1}^n$ and $0 = t_0 < t_1 < t_2 < \ldots < t_n = \tau$. For the sieve approximation, we first choose an appropriate subset $\{\tau_1, \tau_2, \ldots, \tau_m\}$ of $\{t_i\}_1^n$, where τ_j is the terminal point of the jth interval $\mathscr{I}_j = (\tau_{j-1}, \tau_j]$ ($\tau_0 = 0$, $\tau_m = t_n$), such that each $\mathscr{I}_j$ contains nearly an equal number of realizations. We take the following *sieve* approximation of the baseline cumulative hazard $\Lambda_0(t)$:

$$\Lambda_{0m}(t) = \int_0^t \sum_1^m \alpha_i 1\{\tau_{i-1} < u \le \tau_i\}du. \tag{5.11}$$

In this approximation, the sieve parameters $\{\alpha_j\}_1^m$ are the *average hazards* over the associated time intervals $\{\mathscr{I}_j\}_1^m$. By substituting Λ_{0m} into $M_j(t)(j = 1, 2, 3)$, the semiparametric problem is changed into a parametric one.

An algorithm can be used to compute the estimates of β, γ, and $\{\alpha_i\}_1^m$: in the jth step iteration,

$$\Lambda_{0m}^{(j)}(t) = \sum \int_0^t \left[\sum Y_i(u) \exp(\{\beta^{(j-1)} + \gamma^{(j-1)}\}X_i(u))\{\Lambda_{0m}^{(j-1)}(u)\}^{\sigma_i^{(j-1)}-1} \right]^{-1} dN_i(u), \tag{5.12}$$

where

$$\Lambda_{0m}^{(j)}(t), \beta^{(j)}, \quad \gamma^{(j)}, \quad \text{and } \sigma_i^{(j)} = \exp\{\gamma^{(j)}X_i\}$$

denote the jth step iterated values, $j = 0, 1, 2, 3, \ldots$ Initial guess of β and Λ_0 (i.e., $\beta^{(0)}$ and $\Lambda_{0m}^{(0)}$) can be chosen as the estimates of the conventional Cox's model where $\gamma^{(0)} = 0$.

Chapter 6
The Simple Cross-Effect Model

Let $S_X(t)$, $\lambda_X(t)$, and $\Lambda_X(t)$ be the survival, hazard rate, and cumulative hazard functions under a p-dimensional time-dependent covariate X. The generalized proportional hazards (GPH) model proposed by Bagdonavičius and Nikulin (1998a, 1999) holds on a set of explanatory variables E if for all $X \in E$

$$\lambda_X(t) = \psi\{X(t), S_X(t)\}\lambda_0(t). \tag{6.1}$$

This model implies that for different explanatory variables X_1 and X_2 the hazard ratio $HR(t)$ at any moment t is a function of the values $X_1(t)$ and $X_2(t)$ and the probabilities of survival up to t. The proportional hazards model (Cox 1972) is a special case of the GPH model when the function ψ does not depend on $S_X(t)$.

In terms of the cumulative hazard, model (6.1) can be written as

$$\lambda_X(t) = u\{X(t), \Lambda_X(t)\}\lambda_0(t). \tag{6.2}$$

Different choices of $u(\cdot, \cdot)$ lead to submodels with $HR(t)$ increasing or decreasing in time, and cross-effects phenomenon may appear in some cases. We consider here the *cross-effect* model (Bagdonavičius et al. 2004)

$$\lambda_{X(\cdot)}(t) = e^{\beta^T X(t)}\{1 + \Lambda_{X(\cdot)}(t)\}^{1-e^{\gamma^T X(t)}}\lambda_0(t), \tag{6.3}$$

where β and γ are p-dimensional parameters and Λ_0 is an unknown baseline cumulative hazard.

If $X(t) \equiv X$ is constant in time, then resolving a differential equation related to (6.3) and Λ_X produces the *simple cross-effect* (SCE) model:

$$\lambda_X(t) = e^{\beta^T X}\left\{1 + e^{(\beta+\gamma)^T X}\Lambda_0(t)\right\}^{e^{-\gamma^T X}-1}\lambda_0(t), \tag{6.4}$$

where $\Lambda_0(t) = \int_0^t \lambda_0(u)du$ is the baseline cumulative hazard.

© The Author(s) 2016

M. Nikulin and H.-D.I. Wu, *The Cox Model and Its Applications*,
SpringerBriefs in Statistics, DOI 10.1007/978-3-662-49332-8_6

With model (6.4), consider the *hazard ratio*

$$HR(t, X_1, X_2) = \frac{\lambda_{X_2}(t)}{\lambda_{X_1}(t)}, \quad X_1, X_2 \in E_1.$$

At $t = 0$ and under constant covariates X_1 and X_2, assume that $HR(t)$ is greater than 1 and $\gamma^T(X_2 - X_1) > 0$. That is,

$$HR(0, X_1, X_2) = e^{\beta^T(X_2 - X_1)} = c_0 > 1.$$

Then $HR(t)$ decreases from $c_0 > 1$ to 0, indicating that the hazard rates intersect once. The survival functions S_{X_1} and S_{X_2} also intersect once in the interval $(0, \infty)$. The hazards ratio $(HR(t))$ and even the cumulative hazards ratio go to ∞ (or 0) as $t \to 0$; and these ratios are defined and finite at $t = 0$. In pursuit of efficient estimation, this property helps to avoid complexity.

The cross-effect model resembles the extension of the positive stable frailty model (Hougaard 2000) given by Aalen (1992). Indeed, the Hougaard–Aalen model with cross-effects of hazard rates (Aalen 1994) for constant covariates X has one of the two following forms:

$$\lambda_X(t) = \eta r(X)(1 \pm r(X)\alpha^{-1}\delta\eta\Lambda_0(t))^{-\alpha}\lambda_0(t), \quad \alpha, \delta, \eta, r(X) > 0.$$

If we take the minus sign then the hazard rates $\lambda_{X_1}(t)$ and $\lambda_{X_2}(t)$ cross once for constant covariates X_1 and X_2. An unpleasant property of this model is that the survival distributions have finite supports which differ for different covariate values. Estimation procedures are always complicated in such cases. If we take the plus sign and the hazard rates cross for values $\alpha > 1$, the supports are $[0, \infty)$.

The Hougaard–Aalen model also resembles the cross-effect model in that: if we replace the constant α by $1 - e^{-\gamma^T X}$, the function $\eta r(X)$ by $e^{\beta^T X}$, and $\pm r(X)\alpha^{-1}\delta\eta$ by $e^{(\beta+\gamma)^T X}$ in the Hougaard–Aalen model with cross-effects then we obtain the cross-effect model with constant covariates (6.4). Note that in model (6.4) the power $e^{-\gamma^T X} - 1$ can take either sign and the supports of the survival distributions are $[0, \infty)$ for all values of the covariates.

Another difference between the Hougaard–Aalen and the cross-effect models is: the Hougaard–Aalen model includes crossing hazards but not crossing survivals. For the Hougaard–Aalen model, the power α is constant and the survival functions $S_{X_1}(t)$ and $S_{X_2}(t)$ do not cross. For $\alpha \neq 1$ and $r(X_2) > r(X_1)$,

$$\frac{S_{X_2}(t)}{S_{X_1}(t)} = \exp\left\{\frac{\alpha}{\pm\delta(\alpha - 1)}\left[(1 \pm r(X_2)\phi(t))^{1-\alpha} - (1 \pm r(X_1)\phi(t))^{1-\alpha}\right]\right\} < 1,$$

where $\phi(t) = \alpha^{-1}\delta\eta\Lambda_0(t)$; while if $\alpha = 1$, then

$$\frac{S_{X_2}(t)}{S_{X_1}(t)} = \left(\frac{1 - r(X_2)\phi(t)}{1 - r(X_1)\phi(t)}\right)^{\alpha/\delta} < 1.$$

Suppose that model (6.2) holds on a set E_0 of constant explanatory variables. By solving (6.2) in terms of $\Lambda_x(t)$, we have

$$\Lambda_X(t) = H\{X, \Lambda_0(t)\}. \tag{6.5}$$

The Hsieh model takes $H(X, s) = r(X)s^{\rho(X)}$ in (6.5) with natural parameterizations $r(X) = e^{\beta^T X}$ and $\rho(X) = e^{\gamma^T X}$, leading to the PH model if $\gamma = 0$.

Similar to the Hsieh model, the SCE model also gives cross-effect for the cumulative hazards, *not necessarily* for the hazards. When the log HR is of concern, the main differences between these two models are

(I) the Hsieh model assumes that the HR between groups is possibly large when t approaches 0, the SCE model relaxes this assumption; and

(II) in the Hsieh model, HR is increasing or decreasing according to the heteroscedasticity $\gamma^T X$; while the SCE model has more complex situation which depends on the configurations of β and γ in the model formula. Figures 6.1 and 6.2 give

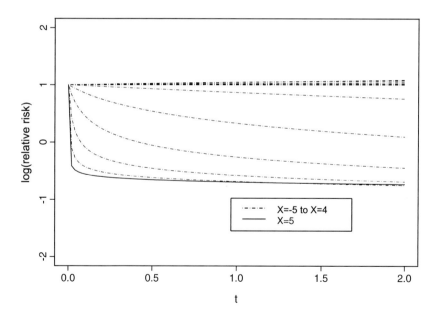

Fig. 6.1 SCE model, gamma $= 0.5$. Reprinted from Probability, Statistics and Modelling in Public Health, H.-D.I. Wu, Statistical Inference for Two-Sample and Regression Models with Heterogeneity Effect: A Collected-Sample Perspective, pp. 452–465, Copyright 2006, with permission from Springer

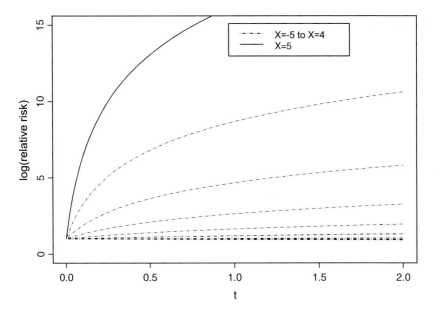

Fig. 6.2 SCE model, gamma $= -0.5$. Reprinted from Probability, Statistics and Modelling in Public Health, H.-D.I. Wu, Statistical Inference for Two-Sample and Regression Models with Heterogeneity Effect: A Collected-Sample Perspective, pp. 452–465, Copyright 2006, with permission from Springer

similar illustrations to Figs. 5.1 and 5.2. When γ is large (0.5 or -0.5), on one hand, the dependence of log HR on t is evident. On the other hand, for larger γ the difference of log HR for different X values is more obvious, showing *heterogeneity* effect over the covariate space. For all cases, we have $\beta = 1$ and $0 < t < 2$.

6.1   Semiparametric Estimation

Consider the GPH model in its general form with a specified parameterization $g(X, s, \theta)$ of the function g via parameters θ and an unknown baseline function $\lambda_0(t)$,

$$\lambda_X(t) = g\{X, \Lambda_0(t), \theta\} \lambda_0(t). \tag{6.6}$$

By the same notations as in Chap. 2, the partial likelihood function (Andersen et al. 1993)

$$L(\theta) = \prod_{i=1}^{n} \left[\int_0^\infty \frac{g\{X_i, \Lambda_0(v), \theta\}}{\sum_{j=1}^{n} Y_j(v) g\{X_j, \Lambda_0(v), \theta\}} \, dN_i(v) \right]^{\delta_i}$$

depends on the unknown cumulative hazard Λ_0. The score function for θ is

$$U(\theta) = \sum_{j=1}^{n} \int_0^\infty \{w^{(i)}(u, \Lambda_0, \theta) - E(u, \Lambda_0, \theta)\} \, dN_i(u), \qquad (6.7)$$

where

$$w^{(i)}(t, \theta, \Lambda_0) = \frac{\partial}{\partial \theta} \log\{g(X_i, \Lambda_0(v), \theta)\},$$

$$E(v, \Lambda_0, \theta) = \frac{S^{(1)}(v, \Lambda_0, \theta)}{S^{(0)}(v, \Lambda_0, \theta)}, \quad S^{(0)}(v, \Lambda_0, \theta) = \sum_{i=1}^{n} Y_i(v) g\{X_i, \Lambda_0(v), \theta\}$$

$$S^{(1)}(v, \Lambda_0, \theta) = \sum_{i=1}^{n} Y_i(v) \frac{\partial}{\partial \theta} g\{X_i, \Lambda_0(v), \theta\}.$$

The score function depends on the unknown function Λ_0, so it is replaced in (6.7) by $\tilde{\Lambda}_0$ (depending on θ) which is defined recurrently from

$$\tilde{\Lambda}_0(t, \theta) = \int_0^t \frac{dN(u)}{S^{(0)}(u-, \tilde{\Lambda}_0, \theta)} \qquad (6.8)$$

This estimator is obtained using the martingale property of the difference,

$$N_i(t) - \int_0^t Y_i(s) d\Lambda_{X_i}(s).$$

The modified score function is

$$\tilde{U}(\theta) = \sum_{j=1}^{n} \int_0^\infty \{w^{(i)}(u, \tilde{\Lambda}_0, \theta) - E(u, \tilde{\Lambda}_0, \theta)\} \, dN_i(u), \qquad (6.9)$$

and the estimators $\hat{\theta}$ and $\hat{\Lambda}_0$ of θ and Λ_0, respectively, satisfy the system of equations

$$\begin{cases} \sum_{j=1}^{n} \int_0^\infty \{w^{(i)}(u, \hat{\Lambda}_0, \hat{\theta}) - E(u, \hat{\Lambda}_0, \hat{\theta})\} \, dN_i(u) = 0, \\ \hat{\Lambda}_0(t) = \tilde{\Lambda}_0(t, \hat{\theta}). \end{cases} \qquad (6.10)$$

Given the consistency of $\tilde{\Lambda}_0$, the asymptotic covariance matrix of $\sqrt{n}(\hat{\theta} - \theta)$ is obtained by standard methods using the *functional delta method* and the *central limit theorem for martingales*. For proof of consistency of the estimators given by Eq. (6.9), see Ceci and Mazliak (2004), Dabrowska (2005–2007). Furthermore, under the current SCE model, the estimator $\hat{\Lambda}_0$ of the baseline cumulative hazard Λ_0

generalizes the Nelson–Aalen estimator, just as in the case of the PH model the
Breslow estimator generalizes the Nelson–Aalen estimator (Andersen et al. 1993).

For the PH model, $g(X, s, \theta) = e^{\theta^T X}$, the solution of the Eqs. (6.10) is $(\hat{\theta}, \hat{\Lambda}_0)$,
where $\hat{\theta}$ is the semiparametrically efficient estimator of the regression parameters θ,
and $\hat{\Lambda}_0$ is the Breslow estimator of Λ_0. This suggests that in the case of the SCE
model,

$$g(X, s, \theta) = e^{\beta^T X} \left\{ 1 + e^{(\beta+\gamma)^T X} s \right\}^{\frac{e^{-\gamma^T X} - 1}{}},$$

the estimator $\hat{\theta}$ also is semiparametrically efficient.

An estimator is semiparametrically efficient if there exists a sequence of parametric models such that the limit covariance matrix of semiparametric estimators
coincides with the limit Fisher information matrix of the sequence of parametric estimators corresponding to the specified models. This should hold in our case because
the parametric score functions obtained by the maximum likelihood method and the
semiparametric score function (6.9) are asymptotically equivalent: the parametric
score function for the model (6.6) is

$$U^*(\theta) = \sum_{j=1}^{n} \int_0^{\infty} \frac{\partial}{\partial \theta} \log \lambda_{X_i}(v, \theta) \{ dN_i(v) - Y_i(v) \lambda_{X_i}(v, \theta) dv \}$$

$$= \sum_{i=1}^{n} \int_0^{\infty} w^{(i)}(u, \Lambda_0, \theta) [dN_i(v) - Y_i(v) g\{X_i, \Lambda_0(v), \theta\} d\Lambda_0(v)]. \quad (6.11)$$

If the function Λ_0 in (6.11) is replaced by $\tilde{\Lambda}_0$ then the modified score function (6.9)
is obtained.

Once the parameter estimators are obtained, the estimator of the survival function
under a specific covariate value $X = x$ is

$$\hat{S}_x(t) = e^{-\hat{\Lambda}_x(t)},$$

where

$$\hat{\Lambda}_x(t) = \left\{ 1 + e^{(\hat{\beta}+\hat{\gamma})^T x} \tilde{\Lambda}_0(t, \theta) \right\}^{\frac{e^{-\hat{\gamma}^T x} - 1}{}}.$$

6.2   An Iterative Procedure for Computing the Estimators

Computationally, it is not necessary to solve (6.9) to obtain the estimate $\hat{\theta}$. Instead,
the general quasi-Newton optimization algorithm can be used to seek the value of θ
which maximizes the modified partial likelihood (MPL) function

$$\tilde{L}(\theta) = \prod_{i=1}^{n} \left[\int_0^{\infty} \frac{g\{x_i, \tilde{\Lambda}_0(v), \theta\}}{\sum_{j=1}^{n} Y_j(v) g\{x_j, \tilde{\Lambda}_0(v), \theta\}} \, dN_i(v) \right]^{\delta_i}. \qquad (6.12)$$

For fixed θ the estimator $\tilde{\Lambda}_0$ can be found as follows. Let $T_1 < \dots < T_r$ be the ordered distinct failure times, $r \le n$, and d_i be the number of failures at T_i. Then

$$\tilde{\Lambda}_0(0; \theta) = 0, \quad \tilde{\Lambda}_0(T_1; \theta) = \frac{d_1}{S^{(0)}(0, \tilde{\Lambda}_0, \theta)},$$

$$\tilde{\Lambda}_0(T_{j+1}; \theta) = \tilde{\Lambda}_0(T_j; \theta) + \frac{d_{j+1}}{S^{(0)}(T_j, \tilde{\Lambda}_0, \theta)}. \quad (j = 1, \dots, r-1) \qquad (6.13)$$

For the SCE model,

$$S^{(0)}(v, \Lambda_0, \theta) = \sum_{i=1}^{n} Y_i(v) \, e^{\beta^T X_i} \{1 + e^{(\beta+\gamma)^T X_i} \Lambda_0(v)\}^{e^{-\gamma^T X_i} - 1},$$

hence

$$\tilde{\Lambda}_0(T_1; \theta) = \frac{d_1}{\sum_{i=1}^{n} Y_i(T_1) \, e^{\beta^T X_i}}.$$

The iterative procedure is very simple. We use the initial value $\theta_0 = (\beta_0, \gamma_0)$, where β_0 is an estimator of β using the PH model, and $\gamma_0 = 1$. Then the estimator $\tilde{\Lambda}(t, \theta_0)$ given by recurrence formula (6.13) and the initial guess θ_0 are plugged into the MPL function (6.12), which we maximize to give θ_1. The value of θ_1 is then used to obtain $\tilde{\Lambda}(t, \theta_1)$ and so on.

6.3 Analysis of Gastric Cancer Data

In this section we give an analysis of the two-sample data of Stablein and Koutrouvelis (1985). The number of patients is 90. Kaplan–Meier (KM) estimators of survival functions pertaining to the both treatment groups (Fig. 1.3 in Chap. 1) clearly show a crossing-effect phenomenon. The two estimated curves indicate that radiotherapy would initially be detrimental to a patient's survival but becomes beneficial later on.

We use the SCE model to estimate the effect of "treatment" (treated as a single covariate) on the survival. The modified partial likelihood estimator of $\theta = (\beta, \gamma)$ is (1.894, 1.384). We use 0 to code for chemotherapy and 1 for chemo- plus radiotherapy. For both groups of patients the graphs of the K–M estimators and the smoothed Hsieh estimators of the survival functions are presented in Fig. 6.3. Smoothing was necessary because the Hsieh estimators are step functions with only five steps (if the number of steps is larger, the estimators of step height may be bad).

Fig. 6.3 K–M estimates and survivals estimated from Hsieh model. Reprinted from Biostatistics, 5(3), V. Bagdonavičius, M.A. Hafdi, M. Nikulin, Analysis of Survival Data with Cross-effects of Survival Functions, p. 125, Copyright 2015, with permission from Oxford

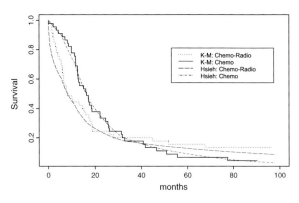

Fig. 6.4 K–M estimates and survivals estimated from SCE model. Reprinted from Biostatistics, 5(3), V. Bagdonavičius, M.A. Hafdi, M. Nikulin, Analysis of Survival Data with Cross-effects of Survival Functions, p. 125, Copyright 2015, with permission from Oxford

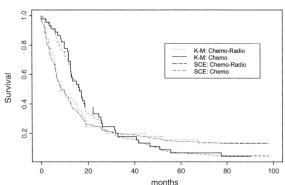

The graphs of the K–M estimators and our estimators of the survival functions are presented in Fig. 6.4. The estimators obtained from all of the data using the regression model (6.4) and our estimation method give excellent fits to the K–M estimators obtained from the two subsamples.

Our estimation procedures should be useful for the analysis with continuously varying covariables, for which the K–M estimators are not applicable.

6.4   Multiple Cross-Effects Model

Another interesting model with cross-effects of survival was proposed by Bagdonavičius and Nikulin (2005, 2006) called *multiple cross-effects* (MCE) model:

$$\lambda_x(t) = e^{\beta^T x} \left(1 + \gamma^T x \Lambda_0(t) + \delta^T x \Lambda_0^2(t)\right) \lambda_0(t), \quad x \in E_1. \qquad (6.14)$$

The regression parameters β, γ, and δ are p-dimensional for this MCE model.

In case one concerns the "homogeneity effect" (or "no lifetime regression"), we can see that it takes place if $\gamma = 0$ and $\beta = 0$ for Hsieh model, $\gamma = 0$ and $\beta = 0$ for SCE model, and $\beta = \delta = \gamma = 0$ for MCE model.

Here we give a brief summary on the properties of the models considered: For the *Hsieh model*, the hazard rates and the survival function do not intersect or intersect once in the interval $(0, \infty)$. For the *SCE model*, the ratio of the hazard rates increase, decrease, or is constant; the hazard rates and the survival function do not intersect or intersect once in the interval $(0, \infty)$. For the *MCE model*, the ratio of the hazard rates increase, decrease, or is constant; the hazard rates and the survival function do not intersect, intersect once or twice in the interval $(0, \infty)$.

Note also that in the case of the GPH model the hazard ratio is increasing, decreasing, or constant in time, the hazard functions and the survival functions do not intersect in the interval $(0, \infty)$.

Finally, for a generalization of the positive stable frailty model given by Aalen (1994),

$$\lambda_x(t) = r(x)\{1 + r(x)\mu^{-1}\delta \Lambda_0(t)\}^\mu \lambda_0(t) \quad (x \in E_1)$$

with $\mu > 1$, the hazard rates intersect but the survival functions do not intersect.

Chapter 7
Goodness-of-Fit for the Cox Model

Goodness-of-fit problem playes a key role in statistical inference because the validity of an assumed model ensures the subsequent inferential rationality. As the Cox PH model,

$$\lambda(t; X) = \lambda_0(t) \exp(\beta^T X),$$

is the most frequently used model in survival analysis, model validation is important for the applications. There are three aspects concerning tests for model validity:

(1) *Omnibus test*: to check for the 'global correctness' of the model. In hypothesis testing language, we are testing for H_0: (the data obeys) Cox model; against H_a: (the data obeys) other models, not Cox model.
(2) *Proportional hazards test*: assuming a wider class (H_a) that contains Cox model as a special case (H_0) and then test for the extra parameter(s).
(3) *Homogeneity test*: Assuming the Cox model or a wider class as the alternative hypothesis (H_a) and then test for suitable parameters for the equality of $K(\geq 2)$ groups.

The advantage of the PH model is its simplicity in interpreting the treatment effect as an instantaneous relative risk adjusted for explanatory covariates. This simplicity, however, constrains applications of the PH model in analyzing survival data in some aspects. For example, when the hazards corresponding to different covariate values *cross* at some points, using Cox's model to estimate the relative risk or using the logrank test to test for group difference may lead to inappropriate conclusions (Breslow et al. 1984; Stablein and Koutrouvelis 1985; Tubert-Bitter et al. 1994; Hsieh 1996).

In contrast to the PH model, there are methods or models proposed to make statistical inference with regards to the crossing hazards phenomenon (Stablein and Koutrouvelis 1985; Moreau et al. 1992). We introduce in Sect. 7.1 several omnibus tests and in Sects. 7.2 and 7.3 how alternative models can be considered to test *proportional hazards* assumption and *homogeneity effect*. At the end, we note that more about tests for model validity for censored and truncated data on can see in Bagdonavicius et al. (2011).

© The Author(s) 2016
M. Nikulin and H.-D.I. Wu, *The Cox Model and Its Applications*,
SpringerBriefs in Statistics, DOI 10.1007/978-3-662-49332-8_7

7.1 Omnibus Tests

Let the partial score process $U_n(t; \beta)$ be obtained by taking partial derivative of
the log partial likelihood process with respect to β (Andersen and Gill 1982), Wei
(1984) introduces a goodness-of-fit approach to the proportional hazards model in
two-sample setting. The process $U_n(t; \widehat{\beta})$, with β replaced by $\widehat{\beta}$, is shown to converge
weakly to a Brownian bridge $W^0(\cdot)$. A natural goodness-of-fit statistic is then the
supremum of $|W^0(\cdot)|$ with suitable scaling, and the distribution of $sup|W^0(\cdot)|$ has
been well studied.

Here we introduce in more details two famous *omnibus* tests for the PH model:
the test of Gill and Schumacher (1987) for two-sample problem and Lin's test for
regression set-up (Lin 1991).

7.1.1 Gill–Schumacher Test

For the considered two samples, let $K(t)$ be a predictable process, τ be a maximal
time of observation, and define

$$Q_K = \int_0^\tau K(t) \left\{ \frac{dN_2(t)}{Y_2(t)} - \frac{dN_1(t)}{Y_1(t)} \right\}.$$

If $\theta \equiv \lambda_2(t)/\lambda_1(t)$ is the hazards ratio (relative risk) of the two groups, then

$$\widehat{\theta}_K = \frac{\int K(t)d\widehat{\Lambda}_2(t)}{\int K(t)d\widehat{\Lambda}_1(t)}$$

is a natural estimate of θ specific to the weight function $K(t)$ and

$$\widehat{\Lambda}_j(t) = \int_0^t \{Y_j(u)\}^{-1} dN_j(u), \quad (j = 1, 2).$$

Under $H_0 : \lambda_1(t) = \lambda_2(t)$, the following two estimates of θ $(\widehat{\theta}_{K_1}$ and $\widehat{\theta}_{K_2})$, which
corresponds to two weight processes K_1 and K_2, will be very close to each other
asymptotically. Or, equivalently, $Q_{GS} = \widehat{K}_{11}\widehat{K}_{22} - \widehat{K}_{12}\widehat{K}_{21}$ should be very close to 0
if $\widehat{K}_{ij}$ is defined as

$$\widehat{K}_{ij} = \int K_i(t)d\widehat{\Lambda}_j(t) \quad (i = 1, 2; j = 1, 2).$$

Gill and Schumacher (1987) proposes the following statistic:

$$T_{GS} = \frac{Q_{GS}}{\sqrt{var(Q_{GS})}}, \tag{7.1}$$

where $var(Q_{GS})$ can be consistently estimated by

$$\widehat{K}_{21}\widehat{K}_{22}\widehat{V}_{11} - \widehat{K}_{21}\widehat{K}_{12}\widehat{V}_{12} - \widehat{K}_{11}\widehat{K}_{22}\widehat{V}_{21} + \widehat{K}_{11}\widehat{K}_{12}\widehat{V}_{22}$$

with

$$\widehat{V}_{ij} = \int K_i(t)K_j(t)\frac{d\{N_1(t) + N_2(t)\}}{Y_1(t)Y_2(t)}.$$

The remaining question is how to choose $K(\cdot)$. Let us consider the class of Fleming–Harrington weight function (K_{FH}) (see Fleming and Harrington 1991 and Harrington and Fleming 1982):

$$K_{FH} = \{\widehat{S}(t)\}^\rho \{1 - \widehat{S}(t)\}^\gamma \frac{Y_1(t)Y_2(t)}{Y_1(t) + Y_2(t)},$$

where $\widehat{S}(t)$ is the Kaplan–Meier estimate of the pooled sample. Possible choice of (ρ, γ) configurations are discussed in Klein and Moeschberger (2003, Chap. 7) and Wu (2007).

7.1.2 Lin Test

For a set of independent copies $(T_i, \delta_i, X_i(t))$ of random samples, let $U_K(\beta)$ be the partial score function derived from logarithm of partial likelihood when a predictable weight process $K(t)$ is imposed:

$$U_K(\beta) = \sum_{i=1}^n \delta_i K(t_i)\left\{X(t_i) - \frac{S^{(1)}(t; \beta)}{S^{(0)}(t; \beta)}\right\},$$

and $\widehat{\beta}_K$ be the solution to $U_K(\beta) = 0$ for $K(t) \neq 1$. When $K(t) = 1$, the solution is denoted as $\widehat{\beta}$ (which is simply the conventional Cox's estimator). Note that, under suitable regularity conditions (Andersen and Gill 1982; Tsiatis 1981), both $\widehat{\beta}_K$ and $\widehat{\beta}$ are consistent estimates of the true parameter β. Lin (1991) shows that,

$$\sqrt{n}(\widehat{\beta}_K - \widehat{\beta}) \sim N(0, \Sigma_K(\beta)),$$

where the asymptotic covariance matrix can be consistently estimated by

$$\Sigma_K(\widehat{\beta}) = C_K^{-1}D_K C_K^{-1} - C_1^{-1},$$

with

$$C_K = \frac{1}{n}\sum \delta_i K(t_i)V(t_i; \widehat{\beta}), \quad D_K = \frac{1}{n}\sum \delta_i K^2(t_i)V(t_i; \widehat{\beta}), \quad C_1 = \frac{1}{n}\sum \delta_i V(t_i; \widehat{\beta}),$$

and

$$V(t; \widehat{\beta}) = \frac{S^{(2)}(t; \beta)}{S^{(0)}(t; \beta)} - \left(\frac{S^{(1)}(t; \beta)}{S^{(0)}(t; \beta)}\right)^{\otimes 2}.$$

Lin's test is constructed as

$$T_{Lin} = (\widehat{\beta}_K - \widehat{\beta})^T \left\{\Sigma_K(\widehat{\beta})\right\}^{-1} (\widehat{\beta}_K - \widehat{\beta}) \sim \chi_p^2, \tag{7.2}$$

where $p = \dim(\beta)$.

7.2 Test for PH Assumption Within a Wider Class

It is common practice to test a hypothesized model (H_0) against a wider class of alternatives (H_a). In linear regressions, for example, t-test can be viewed as testing an extra effect (parameter) with nested model structure; the tested model (H_0) is considered as being nested in the alternative model (H_a) so that the effect of the covariate of main interest is tested. For more than one covariates, the partial F test is used. In logistic regression and Cox's regression, parallel practice leads to Wald test (or score test) with similar spirit of nested model structure. Generally, in survival analysis, testing the validity of a class of models (say, Cox PH model class) can be implemented by the same manner. Here the terminology 'a class of PH models' refers to any Cox's models with proportionality for the collected failure time (T^*), censoring time (C), covariates (X) information and their realizations. A model which does not satisfy the PH model assumption means that the PH model setting is not fulfilled even with the entire (T^*, C, X) information and data realization history. So, constructing a wider class of models (H_a) than the PH-class (H_0) and testing the extra parameter(s) (since PH is nested within the wider class; $H_0 \in H_a$) is appealing. The models and tests considered in Quantin et al. (1996), Bagdonavičius and Nikulin (2011), Wu et al. (2002), and Bagdonavičius et al. (2004), among others, concern this approach with nested models. These more-general models are useful not only for constructing goodness-of-fit tests for the PH assumption and for homogeneity effect, but also for valid estimation and more accurate prediction.

7.2.1 The GPH and SCE Models as Alternative Hypothesis

The generalized proportional hazards (GPH) model and the simple-cross effect (SCE) model has been introduced and discussed in Chap. 6. Based on the modified partial likelihood, both models serve as useful extensions of the PH model. Now we consider how to construct tests based on the modified score functions for the two models.

Let $S_x(t)$, $\lambda_x(t)$ and $\Lambda_x(t)$ be the survival, hazard rate and cumulative hazard functions under a p-dimensional explanatory variable X. Let us consider two models: *Generalized proportional hazards (GPH) model*,

$$\lambda_x(t) = e^{\beta^T x}(1 + \Lambda_x(t))^{-\gamma+1}\lambda(t) = e^{\beta^T x}(1 + \gamma e^{\beta^T x}\Lambda_0(t))^{\frac{1}{\gamma}-1}\lambda_0(t); \qquad (7.3)$$

and *Simple cross-effects (SCE) model*:

$$\lambda_x(t) = e^{\beta^T x}\{1 + \Lambda_x(t)\}^{1-e^{\gamma^T x}}\lambda(t) = e^{\beta^T x}\{1 + e^{(\beta+\gamma)^T x}\Lambda_0(t)\}^{e^{-\gamma^T x}-1}\lambda_0(t). \qquad (7.4)$$

In both models,

$$\Lambda_0(t) = \int_0^t \lambda_0(u)du.$$

The parameter γ is one-dimensional for the GPH model and p-dimensional for the SCE model. The PH is a particular case with $\gamma = 1$ (GPH) or $\gamma = 0$ (SCE). The homogeneity (no lifetime regression) takes place if $\gamma = 1$, $\beta = 0$ (GPH) or $\gamma = 0$, $\beta = 0$ (SCE). In this chapter, we consider the right-censored regression data: $(X_1, \delta_1, x_1), \ldots, (X_n, \delta_n, x_n)$, where X_i is the observed failure time or right-censored time, δ_i is the censoring indicator, and x_i is the covariate(s).

Let us consider tests for checking the adequacy of the PH model

$$H_0 : \lambda_x(t) = e^{\beta^T x}\lambda_0(t)$$

versus the GPH alternative ($\gamma \neq 1$) or the SCE alternative ($\gamma \neq 0$).

For a specified model (GPH or SCE), let $\lambda_i = \lambda_{X_i}(t)$ be the hazard function corresponding to individual i with covariate X_i. The score function is expressed as:

$$U(\theta, \Lambda_0) = \sum_{i=1}^n \int_0^\tau \frac{\partial}{\partial\theta} \log \lambda_i(t, \theta)\{dN_i(t) - Y_i(t)\lambda_i(t, \theta)dt\}, \qquad (7.5)$$

where $\theta = (\beta^T, \gamma^T)^T$ is the column vector of parameters of interest. Denote by $\hat{\beta}$ the maximum partial likelihood estimator of the regression parameter β under the PH model and by $\hat{\Lambda}_0$ the Breslow estimator of the cumulative hazard (see Andersen et al. 1993):

$$\hat{\Lambda}_0(t) = \int_0^t \frac{dN(t)}{S^{(0)}(t, \hat{\beta})}, \quad S^{(0)}(t, \hat{\beta}) = \sum_{l=1}^n Y_l(t)e^{\hat{\beta}^T x_l}. \qquad (7.6)$$

In (7.5), replacing the baseline cumulative hazard Λ_0 by the Breslow estimator, the regression parameter β by $\hat{\beta}$, the parameter γ by $\gamma = 1$ (GPH model) or $\gamma = 0$ (SCE model), we obtain $p + 1$-dimensional and $2p$-dimensional statistics, respectively. The first p components of these statistics are equal to zero. So a one-dimensional

(GPH alternative) or p-dimensional (SCE alternative) statistic $\hat{U}$ is used to obtain the tests. It has the form

$$\hat{U} = \sum_{i=1}^{n} \int_0^\infty \{h(x_i, t, \hat{\beta}) - E_*(t, \hat{\beta})\} dN_i(t),$$

where

$$h(x_i, t, \hat{\beta}) = -\ln(1 + e^{\hat{\beta}^T x_i} \hat{\Lambda}_0(t))$$

for the GPH alternative and

$$h(x_i, t, \hat{\beta}) = -x_i \ln(1 + e^{\hat{\beta}^T x_i} \hat{\Lambda}_0(t))$$

for the SCE alternative. Moreover, in the above expression,

$$E_*(t, \hat{\beta}) = \frac{S_*^{(1)}(t, \hat{\beta})}{S^{(0)}(t, \hat{\beta})},$$

where

$$S_*^{(1)}(t, \hat{\beta}) = -\sum_{l=1}^{n} Y_l(t) e^{\hat{\beta}^T x_l} \ln(1 + e^{\hat{\beta}^T x_l} \hat{\Lambda}_0(t))$$

for the GPH alternative; and

$$S_*^{(1)}(t, \hat{\beta}) = -\sum_{l=1}^{n} x_l Y_l(t) e^{\hat{\beta}^T x_l} \ln(1 + e^{\hat{\beta}^T x_l} \hat{\Lambda}_0(t))$$

for the SCE alternative.

It can be shown that (when $k = 1$ for the GPH alternative and $k = p$ for the SCE alternative),

$$T = n^{-1} \hat{U}^T \hat{D}^{-1} \hat{U} \xrightarrow{\mathcal{D}} \chi^2(k),$$

where

$$\hat{D} = \hat{\Sigma}_{**} - \hat{\Sigma}_*^T \hat{\Sigma}_0^{-1} \hat{\Sigma}_*,$$

with

$$\hat{\Sigma}_* = \frac{1}{n} \sum_{i:\delta_i=1} V_*(X_i, \hat{\beta}), \quad \hat{\Sigma}_{**} = \frac{1}{n} \sum_{i:\delta_i=1} V_{**}(X_i, \hat{\beta}),$$

and

$$\hat{\Sigma}_0 = \frac{1}{n} \sum_{i:\delta_i=1} \left\{ \frac{S^{(2)}(X_i; \hat{\beta})}{S^{(0)}(X_i; \hat{\beta})} - \left(\frac{S^{(1)}(X_i; \hat{\beta})}{S^{(0)}(X_i; \hat{\beta})} \right)^{\otimes 2} \right\}.$$

In these expressions,

$$V_*(u, \hat{\beta}) = \frac{S_*^{(2)}(u, \hat{\beta})}{S^{(0)}(u, \hat{\beta})} - E(u, \hat{\beta})E_*^T(u, \hat{\beta}), \qquad (7.7)$$

$$V_{**}(u, \hat{\beta}) = \frac{S_{**}^{(2)}(u, \hat{\beta})}{S^{(0)}(u, \hat{\beta})} - E_*^{\otimes 2}(u, \hat{\beta}). \qquad (7.8)$$

Moreover, for the GPH model,

$$S_*^{(2)}(u, \hat{\beta}) = -\sum_{l=1}^{n} x_l Y_l(t) e^{\hat{\beta}^T x_l} \ln(1 + e^{\hat{\beta}^T x_l} \hat{\Lambda}_0(t)),$$

$$S_{**}^{(2)}(u, \hat{\beta}) = -\sum_{l=1}^{n} Y_l(t) e^{\hat{\beta}^T x_l} \ln^2(1 + e^{\hat{\beta}^T x_l} \hat{\Lambda}_0(t)); \qquad (7.9)$$

for the SCE model,

$$S_*^{(2)}(u, \hat{\beta}) = -\sum_{l=1}^{n} x_l^{\otimes 2} Y_l(t) e^{\hat{\beta}^T x_l} \ln(1 + e^{\hat{\beta}^T x_l} \hat{\Lambda}_0(t)),$$

$$S_{**}^{(2)}(u, \hat{\beta}) = -\sum_{l=1}^{n} x_l^{\otimes 2} Y_l(t) e^{\hat{\beta}^T x_l} \ln^2(1 + e^{\hat{\beta}^T x_l} \hat{\Lambda}_0(t)). \qquad (7.10)$$

The null hypothesis is rejected with the significance level α if $T > \chi_{1-\alpha}^2(k)$.

7.2.2 The Hsieh Model as an Alternative

Consider the Hsieh (2001) model introduced in Sect. 5.4 and use the same notations. Define a covariation process $A(t)$, which is a matrix with components (Andersen et al. 1993)

$$A_{ij} = \lim \frac{1}{n} \sum \int E\{dM_i(u)\}\{dM_j(u)\}du.$$

Further, let $\hat{M}_j = M_j(\hat{\theta}, \hat{\Lambda}_0), j = 2, 3$; and

$$\hat{A}_{ij} = \frac{1}{n} \sum \int E\{d\hat{M}_i(u)\}\{d\hat{M}_j(u)\}du.$$

Using the estimates $(\hat{\theta}, \hat{\Lambda}_0)$ obtained from some numerical algorithms and treating M_2 and M_3 as score functions of β and γ, respectively, the following two statistics (T_W and T_S), evaluated at $(\beta, \gamma; \Lambda_0) = (\hat{\beta}, 0; \hat{\Lambda}_0)$ and $t = \tau$ (the maximal observation time), can be used to test the null hypothesis $H_0 : \gamma = 0$:

$$T_W = \{\sqrt{n}\hat{\gamma}\}^T \{\hat{A}_{33} - \hat{A}_{32}\hat{A}_{22}^{-1}\hat{A}_{23}\}\{\sqrt{n}\hat{\gamma}\}, \tag{7.11}$$

which is a Wald-type statistic, and

$$T_S = \{M_3\}^T \{M^{\gamma\gamma}\}\{M_3\}, \tag{7.12}$$

a score-type statistic. In (7.12)

$$M^{\gamma\gamma} = -\{M_{33} - M_{32}^T M_{22}^{-1} M_{23}\}^{-1},$$

where

$$M_{22} = \partial M_2/\partial\beta, \quad M_{23} = \partial M_2/\partial\gamma, \quad \text{and} \quad M_{33} = \partial M_3/\partial\gamma.$$

Under H_0, both T_W and T_S have asymptotically a χ_1^2 distribution.

7.3 Test for Homogeneity Within a Wider Class: Two-Sample Problem

Two-sample tests for the hypothesis of the equality of two distributions from censored samples were considered, for examples, by Koziol (1978), Peto and Peto (1972), Tarone and Ware (1977), Aalen (1992), Kalbfleisch and Prentice (2002), Fleming and Harrington (1991), and Harrington and Fleming (1982). The classical weighted logrank tests have unsatisfactory power under the alternative of crossing survival functions because early differences in favor of one group are negated by late survival advantage of another group. Stablein and Koutrouvelis (1985), Bagdonavičius et al. (2004, 2011) considered tests for equality of survival distributions against the alternative of single crossing of survival functions. Here we consider a test against general classes of alternatives including the GPH and SCE models.

7.3.1 GPH and SCE Models

Consider the univariate case when X is the only "covariate" and it is dichotomous ($X = 1$ denotes the first group and $X = 0$ the second group), then we have a *two-sample problem*. In such a case we use the following notation. Denote by n_i the sample size of the *i*th group ($i = 1, 2$). Denote by T_{ij}^* and C_{ij} the failure and censoring times for the *j*th object of the *i*th group, and set

$$T_{ij} = \min(T_{ij}^*, C_{ij}), \quad \delta_i = 1_{\{T_{ij}^* \leq C_{ij}\}},$$

$$N_{ij}(t) = 1_{\{T_{ij}^* \leq t, \delta_{ij} = 1\}}, \quad Y_{ij}(t) = 1_{\{T_{ij} \geq t\}}.$$

Moreover,

$$N_{i\cdot}(t) = \sum_{j=1}^{n_i} N_{ij}(t), \quad Y_{i\cdot}(t) = \sum_{j=1}^{n_i} Y_{ij}(t),$$

$$N(t) = N_{1\cdot}(t) + N_{2\cdot}(t), \quad Y(t) = Y_{1\cdot}(t) + Y_{2\cdot}(t).$$

The homogeneity hypothesis is

$$H_0 : F_1 = F_2,$$

where F_i is the distribution function of the units of the *i*th group. The alternatives are GPH with $(\beta, \gamma) \neq (0, 1)$ or SCE with $(\beta, \gamma) \neq (0, 0)$.

Replacing the cumulative hazard Λ by the Nelson–Aalen estimator

$$\hat{\Lambda}(t) = \int_0^t \frac{dN(t)}{Y(t)},$$

the parameters β, γ by $\beta = 0, \gamma = 1$ (GPH model), $\gamma = 0$ (GPH and SCE models) in the score function (7.5), we obtain the statistic

$$\hat{U} = \sum_{i=1}^n \int_0^\infty h(x_i, t)\{dN_i(t) - Y_i(t)d\hat{\Lambda}(t)\}$$

$$= \int_0^\infty \varphi(t) \left(\frac{Y_{2\cdot}(t)}{Y(t)} dN_{1\cdot}(t) - \frac{Y_{1\cdot}(t)}{Y(t)} dN_{2\cdot}(t) \right);$$

here $\varphi(t) = h(1, t) - h(0, t)$.

(a) For the GPH model:

$$h(x, t) = (h_1(x), h_2(x, t)) = (x, -\ln(1 + \hat{\Lambda}(t)), \quad \varphi(t) = (\varphi_1(t), \varphi_2(t)) = (1, 0).$$

(b) For the SCE model:

$$h(x, t) = (h_1(x), h_2(x, t)) = (x, -x\ln(1 + \hat{\Lambda}(t))),$$

$$\varphi(t) = (\varphi_1(t), \varphi_2(t)) = (1, -\ln(1 + \hat{\Lambda}(t))).$$

For both GPH and SCE models, $\hat{U} = (\hat{U}_1, \hat{U}_2)$. In the case of the GPH model, the second component $\hat{U}_2 = 0$ and so $\hat{U} = \hat{U}_1$. The statistic $\hat{U}$ is one- or two-dimensional when it is obtained using the GPH or SCE model, respectively.

The jth component $\hat{U}_j$ of the statistic $\hat{U}$ can be written as:

$$\hat{U}_j = \int_0^\infty \varphi_j(t) \left(\frac{Y_{2\cdot}(t)}{Y(t)} dN_{1\cdot}(t) - \frac{Y_{1\cdot}(t)}{Y(t)} dN_{2\cdot}(t) \right).$$

Each component is a logrank-type statistic. So in the case of the GPH model we do not obtain anything new except for the usual logrank statistic. It works well against the GPH alternative. It is more interesting for the case of the SCE model. To obtain powerful tests against this alternative, a two-dimensional vector of logrank-type statistics with specified weights are needed.

The statistics $\hat{U}_j(t)$ are local martingales with respect to the history generated by the data (Andersen et al. 1993) and the limit distribution of the statistic $\hat{U}$ is obtained similarly as the limit distribution of univariate logrank-type statistics using the martingale central limit theorem and the fact that the predictable covariations are

$$< \hat{U}_j, \hat{U}_{j'} > (t) = \int_0^t \varphi_j(t)\varphi_{j'}(t) \frac{Y_{1\cdot}(t)Y_2(t)}{Y(t)} d\Lambda(t).$$

The distribution of the statistic $\hat{U}$ is approximated by the normal law $N(0, \Sigma)$ with the covariance matrix being estimated by $\hat{\Sigma} = || \hat{\sigma}_{jj'} ||$,

$$\hat{\sigma}_{jj'} = \int_0^\infty \varphi_j(t)\varphi_{j'}(t) \frac{Y_{1\cdot}(t)Y_{2\cdot}(t)}{Y^2(t)} dN(t).$$

The matrix $\hat{\Sigma}$ is 2×2 when the alternative is the SCE model. Under null hypothesis the law of the statistic

$$X^2 = \hat{U}^T \hat{\Sigma}^{-1} \hat{U}$$

is approximated by χ_2^2 distribution. The null hypothesis is rejected with the significance level α if $X^2 > \chi_{1-\alpha}^2(2)$, where $\chi_{1-\alpha}^2(2)$ is the $(1 - \alpha)$-quantile of χ_2^2 distribution.

It should be noted that when X contains a one-dimensional treatment variable (corresponds to β) and a p-dimensional covariate (corresponds to γ), then the above X^2 statistic can be adequately amended so that it will have a χ_{p+1}^2 distribution (see Examples 4 and 5 below).

7.3.2 The Hsieh Model

When *non-proportional hazards* is present, partial likelihood inference based on the PH model leads to a biased estimate of the *hazard ratio* specific to the treatment or a covariate (Wu 2004). The weighted logrank tests are capable of dealing with this case (Gill 1980; Harrington and Fleming 1982; Moreau et al. 1992). In particular, Fleming and Harrington (1991, Chap. 7) presented a class of $G^{\rho,\gamma}$-statistic so that different weights are used to emphasize early-, middle-, or late-stage differences.

Assume the null hypothesis ($\mathcal{H}_0$) that the hazards of different groups are equal, and take the *Hsieh model* as an alternative ($\mathcal{H}_a$). Let $N_i(t)$ be the counting process of individual i associated with the intensity

$$h_i(t) = Y_i(t)\lambda_0(t)\exp\{(\beta+\phi)'X_i(t)\}\{\Lambda_0(t)\}^{\exp(\phi'X_i(t))-1},$$

and

$$S_J(t) = \frac{1}{n}\sum Y_i(t)J_i(t)\exp\{(\beta+\phi)'X_i(t)\}\{\Lambda_0(t)\}^{\exp(\phi'X_i(t))-1},$$

for a predictable process $J(t)$, $J(t) = 1$, $X(t)$, or $V(t)$ where

$$V_i(t) = X_i(t)\exp(\gamma^T X_i)\log\{\Lambda_0(t)\}.$$

For a maximal observation time τ, $\theta = (\beta^T, \gamma^T)^T$. We have the $\sqrt{n}$-scaled estimating functions for β and γ:

$$E_\beta = \frac{1}{\sqrt{n}}\sum\int_0^t \{X_i(u) - \frac{S_X(u; \Lambda_0, \theta)}{S_1(u; \Lambda_0, \theta)}\}dN_i(u), \qquad (7.14)$$

$$E_\gamma = \frac{1}{\sqrt{n}}\sum\int_0^t \{V_i(u) - \frac{S_V(u; \Lambda_0, \theta)}{S_1(u; \Lambda_0, \theta)}\}dN_i(u); \qquad (7.15)$$

along with the piecewise-constant approximation $\Lambda_{0m}(t)$.

Assuming the Hsieh model in the current problem, the null hypothesis is $\mathcal{H}_0$: $\beta = \gamma = 0$; and the alternative is $\mathcal{H}_a$: β and γ are both arbitrary and finite. A score-type test statistic can be constructed as

$$\mathcal{W} = \{E_\beta, E_\gamma\}\mathcal{I}^{-1}\{E_\beta, E_\gamma\}^T, \qquad (7.18)$$

evaluated at $(\beta, \gamma, \Lambda_0(\tau)) = (0, 0, \widehat{\Lambda}_0(\tau))$. The information matrix, $\mathcal{I}$, defined as

$$\mathcal{I} = \begin{pmatrix} \mathcal{I}_{\beta\beta} & \mathcal{I}_{\beta\gamma} \\ \mathcal{I}_{\gamma\beta} & \mathcal{I}_{\gamma\gamma} \end{pmatrix},$$

has the components

$$\mathcal{I}_{\beta\beta} = \frac{1}{n}\sum\int_0^\tau \{X_i - \frac{S_X(u; \Lambda_0, \theta)}{S_1(u; \Lambda_0, \theta)}\}^{\otimes 2}dN_i(u),$$

$$\mathscr{I}_{\gamma\gamma} = \frac{1}{n} \sum \int_0^\tau \{V_i - \frac{S_V(u; \Lambda_0, \theta)}{S_1(u; \Lambda_0, \theta)}\}^{\otimes 2} dN_i(u),$$

and

$$\mathscr{I}_{\beta\gamma} = \mathscr{I}_{\gamma\beta} = \frac{1}{n} \sum \int_0^\tau \{X_i - \frac{S_X(u; \Lambda_0, \theta)}{S_1(u; \Lambda_0, \theta)}\}\{V_i - \frac{S_V(u; \Lambda_0, \theta)}{S_1(u; \Lambda_0, \theta)}\} dN_i(u).$$

The score statistic $\mathscr{W}$ is asymptotically distributed as χ^2_{2p} under H_0 and $p = dim(X)$.

For the two-sample case studied in Wu (2007), assume that a person stays in the same group throughout the study. Let $\mathscr{D}_{ji}$ be the number of failures in group j ($j = 0, 1$) at time t_i. Assuming no ties, $\mathscr{D}_{1i} = 1$ if the individual who failed is a member of group 1 and $\mathscr{D}_{1i} = 0$ otherwise. Further, $\overline{Y}_{ji}$ is the risk set size of group j at time t_i. Under H_0, $\lambda_1 = \lambda_0$, the estimating functions reduce to

$$E_\beta = \frac{1}{\sqrt{n}} \sum (\mathscr{D}_{1i} - \mathscr{E}_{1i}) \text{ and } E_\gamma = \frac{1}{\sqrt{n}} \sum \Delta_i (\mathscr{D}_{1i} - \mathscr{E}_{1i}), \tag{7.19}$$

where $\Delta_i = \log \Lambda_0(t_i)$; and $\mathscr{E}_{1i} = \overline{Y}_{1i}/\overline{Y}_i, \overline{Y}_i = \overline{Y}_{1i} + \overline{Y}_{0i}$, is the probability calculated at t_i when the failed person belongs to group 1. The information matrix has the elements:

$$\mathscr{I}_{\beta\beta} = \frac{1}{n} \sum (\mathscr{D}_{1i} - \mathscr{E}_{1i})^2, \quad \mathscr{I}_{\beta\gamma} = \frac{1}{n} \sum \Delta_i (\mathscr{D}_{1i} - \mathscr{E}_{1i})^2, \text{ and } \mathscr{I}_{\gamma\gamma} = \frac{1}{n} \sum \Delta_i^2 (\mathscr{D}_{1i} - \mathscr{E}_{1i})^2. \tag{7.20}$$

In these expressions, Δ_i can be substituted by $\widehat{\Delta}_i = \log \widehat{\Lambda}_0(t_i)$. Another simpler choice for estimating $\Lambda_0(t)$ is $\widetilde{\Lambda}_0(t) = \sum_{k \leq i}\{\overline{Y}_k\}^{-1}$. We denote the proposed $\mathscr{W}$ statistic as $\mathscr{W}_A$ and $\mathscr{W}_0$ when $\widehat{\Lambda}_0(t_i)$ and $\widetilde{\Lambda}_0(t_i)$ are used, respectively.

The $\mathscr{W}$-statistic in (7.18) is distributed as χ^2_2 under $\mathscr{H}_0$ because, in two-sample setting, $\dim(X) = 1$. The performance of $\mathscr{W}$ is comparable to a class of weighted logrank tests $G^{\rho,\gamma}$ (Fleming and Harrington 1991, Chap. 7):

$$T_{\mathscr{K}} = \frac{\{\sum_1^n \mathscr{K}(t_i)(\mathscr{D}_{1i} - \mathscr{E}_{1i})\}^2}{\sum_1^n \mathscr{K}^2(t_i)\mathscr{E}_{1i}(1 - \mathscr{E}_{1i})} \tag{7.21}$$

for the choice of weight process:

$$\mathscr{K}(t_i) = \{\widehat{S}(t_i-)\}^\rho \{1 - \widehat{S}(t_i-)\}^\gamma.$$

The quantity $\widehat{S}(t-)$ is the Kaplan–Meier estimate of survival function of the *pooled sample*. Here, note that $G^{0,0}$-statistic corresponds to the "ordinary" logrank statistic and $G^{1,0}$ to the Wilcoxon–Peto–Prentice statistic.

7.3.3   Examples

Example 1 (for Hsieh model): The data analyzed in Stablein and Koutrouvelis (1985) and Hsieh (2001) concerning gastric cancers, and the data listed in Piantadosi (1997, Chap. 19, pp. 483–488) concerning the survival times of lung cancer patients are used to illustrate the implementation of the $\mathscr{W}$-statistics, compared with $G^{\rho,\gamma}$ statistics. The following table gives the results of the tests. Reprinted from Journal of Statistical Planning and Inference, 137(2), H.-D.I. Wu, A Partial Score Test for Difference Among Heterogeneous Populations, pp. 527–537, Copyright 2015, with permission from Elsevier.

Test	$G^{0,0}$	$G^{1,0}$	$G^{1,1}$	$G^{0,1}$	$\mathscr{W}_A$	$\mathscr{W}_0$
Gastric cancer						
Realization	0.222	3.963	0.015	2.071	7.941	10.472
(*p*-value)	(0.637)	(0.046)	(0.902)	(0.150)	(0.019)	(0.005)
Lung cancer						
Realization	1.275	3.177	0.349	0.001	6.394	5.714
(*p*-value)	(0.259)	(0.075)	(0.555)	(0.994)	(0.041)	(0.057)

Gastric cancer data: There were 90 patients randomized into two groups, each had 45 individuals receiving chemotherapy and chemo-plus radiotherapy. A cross point appeared at around 32 months between the two groups (Fig. 1.3.) The *p*-values of the $G^{1,1}$- and $G^{0,1}$-tests are 0.902 and 0.150, respectively. The $G^{1,0}$-test and the tests $\mathscr{W}_A$ and $\mathscr{W}_0$, give significant results of testing for the group difference at the 0.05 nominal level. When the Hsieh model is applied, we have $(\hat{\beta}, \hat{\gamma}) = (0.3251, -0.7933)$ with corresponding *p*-values 0.3267 and 0.0559.

Lung cancer data: There were 164 patients divided into two groups; 86 received radiotherapy and 78 received radiotherapy plus "CAP". We observe from Fig. 1.5 that the Kaplan–Meier estimates cross at around 33 months. The performance of $G^{0,1}$ (putting weight on the late stage) and $G^{1,1}$ (putting weight on middle stage) are both poor at detecting the difference (*p*-value $= 0.994$ and 0.555). However, the $G^{1,0}$-test has a *p*-value of 0.075; the $\mathscr{W}$'s yield smaller significance probabilities than the $G^{\rho,\gamma}$-statistic does. Under the Hsieh model, $(\hat{\beta}, \hat{\gamma}) = (0.2781, -0.4914)$ have *p*-values 0.181 and 0.085. The $\mathscr{W}_A$ test is significant with *p*-value $= 0.041$; and $\mathscr{W}_0$-test gives a *p*-value of 0.057. In Figs. 7.1, 7.2 and 7.3, we present the fits of survival estimates based on Cox's model (Fig. 7.1), Hsieh model (Fig. 7.2), and the SCE model (Fig. 7.3). Cox model certainly does not have good fits for this data due to the cross effect; Hsieh model can capture Group B at the early stage (time $<$ 23 months) and capture Group A at the middle stage (time $>$ 15 months). The SCE model offers smoother estimates that can fit better for almost the entire graph.

Example 2 (for GPH model): The survival data of 137 lung cancer patients given in Kalbfleisch and Prentice (2002) shows that the hazard rates under different values of the covariate (performance status) do not intersect but the ratios of hazard rates

Fig. 7.1 Compare KM and
Cox estimates for lung
cancer data

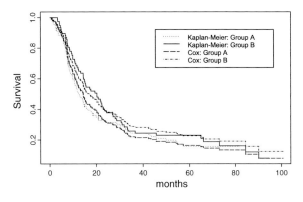

Fig. 7.2 Compare KM and
Hsieh estimates for lung
cancer data. Reprinted from
Journal of Statistical
Planning and Inference,
137(2), H.-D.I. Wu, A Partial
Score Test for Difference
Among Heterogeneous
Populations, pp. 527–537,
Copyright 2015, with
permission from Elsevier

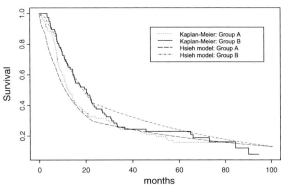

Fig. 7.3 Compare KM and
SCE estimates for lung
cancer data

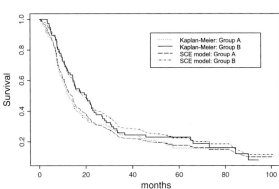

are monotone. So, we apply the test for the Cox model when the alternative is the GPH model. Nine observations were censored, i.e., the proportion of censorings is 0.0657.

Performance status is determined by the Karnofsky index values: 10–30 completely hospitalized, 40–60 partial confinement, 70–90 able to care for self. We used the following models for the analysis:

(a) Continuous covariate *per* (performance status).
(b) Covariate $\mathbf{1}_{\{perf \leq 50\}}$ (performance status dichotomised).

The goodness-of-fit test for the PH against the GPH model was used for these two cases. The test statistic T equals to 8.156 (case a, p-value $= 0.0043$) and 8.563 (case b, p-value $= 0.0034$), respectively. So the PH model is rejected.

In the case of dichotomous covariable, the estimators of the survival functions (corresponding to 0 and 1 performance status) obtained from the GPH model are much closer to the Kaplan–Meier estimates than the estimates obtained from the PH model (Bagdonavičius et al. 2002).

Example 3 (for SCE): The survival data of 90 gastric cancer patients (Example 3, Chap. 1) given in Stablein and Koutrouvelis (1985) concerned the effects of chemotherapy (sample size of 45; treatment indicator $Z = 0$) and chemotherapy plus radiotherapy (sample size of 45; treatment indicator $Z = 1$) on the survival shows that the Kaplan–Meier estimators pertaining to the both treatment groups cross once (Fig. 1.3). We apply the test for the Cox model when the alternative is the SCE model. In this example, eight observations were censored (censoring proportion $= 0.0889$).

The distribution of the test statistic is approximated by the chi-square distribution with one degree of freedom and its value is $T = 13.131$ (p-value $= 0, 0002$). The proportional hazards hypothesis is strongly rejected.

We applied the SCE model for estimation of the influence of covariates to the survival. The modified partial likelihood estimator of $\theta = (\beta, \gamma)$ is (1.8945, 1.3844). The estimators of the survival functions cross at about $t_0 = 28$ (months). The resulting inference indicates that the radiotherapy would first be detrimental to a patient's survival but becomes beneficial later on. Unfortunately, only about 20 % patients survived beyond the time t_0.

Example 4. To illustrate the application of the proposed test for models with more than one covariate we begin with right-censored UIS data set given by Hosmer et al. (2008).

UIS was a 5-year research project comprised two concurrent randomized trials of residential treatment for drug abuse. The purpose of the study was to compare treatment programs of different planned durations designed to reduce drug abuse and to prevent high-risk HIV behavior. The UIS sought to determine whether alternative residential treatment approaches are variable in effectiveness and whether efficacy depends on planned program duration. The time variable is time to return to drug use (measured from admission). The individuals who did not return to drug use are right-censored. We use the model with 10 covariates (which support PH assumption) given by Hosmer, Lemeshow and May (2008). The covariates are: age (years); Beck depression score (becktota; 0–54); $NDRUGFP1 = ((NDRUGTX + 1)/10) ** (-1)$;

Table 7.1 The estimated coefficients

Covariate	DF	Parameter estimate	Standard error	Chi-Square	Pr > ChiSq	Hazard ratio
AGE	1	−0.04140	0.00991	17.4395	<0.0001	0.959
becktota	1	0.00874	0.00497	3.0968	0.0784	1.009
NDRUGFP1	1	−0.57446	0.12519	21.0567	<0.0001	0.563
NDRUGFP2	1	−0.21458	0.04859	19.5043	<0.0001	0.807
IVHX_3	1	0.22775	0.10856	4.4009	0.0359	1.256
RACE	1	−0.46689	0.13476	12.0039	0.0005	0.627
TREAT	1	−0.24676	0.09434	6.8416	0.0089	0.781
SITE	1	−1.31699	0.53144	6.1412	0.0132	0.268
AGEXSITE	1	0.03240	0.01608	4.0596	0.0439	1.033
RACEXSITE	1	0.85028	0.24776	11.7778	0.0006	2.340

$NDRUGFP2 = ((NDRUGTX+1)/10)**(-1)*log((NDRUGTX+1)/10)$; drug use history at admission (IVHX_3; 1—recent, 0—never or previous); race (0—white, 1—non-white); treatment randomization assignment (treat; 0—short, 1—Long); treatment site (site; 0—A, 1—B); interaction of age and treatment site (agexsite); interaction of race and treatment site (racexsite). The NDRUGTX denotes number of prior drug treatments (0–40). Due to missing data in covariates, the model is based on 575 of the 628 observations. The estimated coefficients β are given in Table 7.1.

The value of the test statistic T is 13.3885, the p-value is 0.2028 (because T is now distributed as χ^2_{10}). The assumption of Cox model is not rejected. Note that this example parallels the overall F-test in a conventional multiple linear regression.

Example 5. The data given in Kleinbaum and Klein (2005) are reported from a study in which two methadone treatment clinics for heroin addicts were compared to assess the time of patients that remained under methadone treatment. The variable "time" (in days) is the time until the person dropped out of the clinic or was righted censored. The covariates are prison—indicates whether the patient had a prison record (coded as 1) or not (coded as 0); dose—the continuous variable for the patient maximum methadone dose (mg/day); clinic—indicates which methadone treatment clinic the patient attended (coded as 1 or 2). The value of test statistic T ($\sim\chi^2_3$) is 13.02 with p-value 0.0046. The assumption of the Cox model is rejected. The method based on Schoenfeld (1980) residuals (not reported here) yields the same conclusion.

7.4   Goodness-of-Fit for the Cox Model from Left Truncated and Right-Censored Data

In this section, we consider general tests based on modified score functions obtained from *left truncated and right-censored* data. Let $S_z(t)$, $\lambda_z(t)$ and $\Lambda_z(t)$ be the survival, hazard rate, and cumulative hazard functions under a p-dimensional explanatory variable z. The null hypothesis is the Cox model:

$$H_0 : \ \lambda_z(t) = e^{\beta^T z} \lambda_0(t);$$

where $\lambda_0(t)$ is unknown baseline hazard function, the parameter β is p-dimensional.

Let us consider the SCE model introduced in a previous context. The Cox model is obtained by taking $\gamma = 0$. So, the alternative H_a is the model (4) with $\gamma \neq 0$.

Suppose that survival distributions of all n objects given x_i are absolutely continuous with the survival functions $S_i(t)$ and the hazard rates $\lambda_i(t)$, and the truncation and censoring are non-informative (see Andersen et al. 1993; Huber et al. 2006; Solev 2009; Turnbull 1976). Assume the multiplicative intensities model, the compensator of the counting processes N_i with respect to the history of the observed processes is $\int Y_i \lambda_i du$.

In the parametric case with known λ_0, the unknown finite-dimensional parameter $\theta = (\beta, \gamma)$. The parametric maximum likelihood (ML) estimator $\hat{\theta}$ of the parameter θ satisfies the equation: $\dot{\ell}(\theta; \Lambda) = 0$, where the score function $\dot{\ell}(\theta; \Lambda) = (\dot{\ell}_\beta(\theta; \Lambda), \dot{\ell}_\gamma(\theta; \Lambda))^T$ has the following components:

$$\dot{\ell}_\beta(\theta; \Lambda_0) = \sum_{i=1}^{n} \int_0^\infty \left(z_i + (e^{-\gamma^T z_i} - 1) \frac{z_i e^{(\beta+\gamma)^T z_i} \Lambda_0(t)}{1 + e^{(\beta+\gamma)^T z_i} \Lambda_0(t)} \right)$$
$$\times \{ dN_i(t) - Y_i(t) e^{\beta^T z_i} \{1 + e^{(\beta+\gamma)^T z_i} \Lambda_0(t)\}^{e^{-\gamma^T z_i} - 1} d\Lambda_0(t) \},$$

$$\dot{\ell}_\gamma(\theta; \Lambda_0) = \sum_{i=1}^{n} \int_0^\infty \left(-z_i e^{-\gamma^T z_i} \ln \left[1 + e^{(\beta+\gamma)^T z_i} \Lambda_0(t) \right] + (e^{-\gamma^T z_i} - 1) \frac{z_i e^{(\beta+\gamma)^T z_i} \Lambda_0(t)}{1 + e^{(\beta+\gamma)^T z_i} \Lambda_0(t)} \right)$$
$$\times \{ dN_i(t) - Y_i(t) e^{\beta^T z_i} \{1 + e^{(\beta+\gamma)^T z_i} \Lambda_0(t)\}^{e^{-\gamma^T z_i} - 1} d\Lambda_0(t) \}.$$

Let us consider the case of unknown baseline hazard λ_0. The idea of test construction is simple. In the expression of $\dot{\ell}(\theta; \Lambda_0)$ the parameter γ is replaced by 0, the parameter β by its estimator $\hat{\beta}$ obtained from maximizing the partial likelihood function under the Cox model; i.e., $\hat{\beta}$ satisfies the equation

$$\dot{\ell}(\beta) = \sum_{i=1}^{n} \int_0^\infty \{ z_i - E(t, \beta) \} dN_i(t),$$

where

$$E(t, \beta) = \frac{S^{(1)}(t, \beta)}{S^{(0)}(t, \beta)}, \quad S^{(0)}(t, \beta) = \sum_{i=1}^{n} Y_i(t) e^{\beta^T z_i}, \quad S^{(1)}(t, \beta) = \sum_{i=1}^{n} z_i Y_i(t) e^{\beta^T z_i}.$$

The baseline cumulative intensity Λ_0 is replaced by the Breslow estimator (see Andersen et al. 1993):

$$\hat{\Lambda}_0(t) = \int_0^t \frac{dN(t)}{S^{(0)}(t, \hat{\beta})} = \sum_{i=1}^n Y_i(t)e^{\hat{\beta}^T z_i}.$$

Note that

$$\dot{\ell}_\beta(\hat{\beta}, 0; \hat{\Lambda}_0) = \sum_{i=1}^n \int_0^\infty z_i\{dN_i(t) - Y_i(t)e^{\hat{\beta}^T z_i} d\hat{\Lambda}_0(t)\} = \sum_{i=1}^n \int_0^\infty \{z_i - E(t, \hat{\beta})\}dN_i(t),$$

which equals to 0. We use only the statistic

$$U = \dot{\ell}_\gamma(\hat{\beta}, 0; \hat{\Lambda}_0),$$

which can be written in the form $U = U(\infty)$, where

$$U(t) = -\sum_{i=1}^n \int_0^t z_i \ln\left[1 + e^{\hat{\beta}^T z_i} \hat{\Lambda}_0(t)\right] \{dN_i(t) - Y_i(t)e^{\hat{\beta}^T z_i} d\hat{\Lambda}_0(t)\}$$

$$= \sum_{i=1}^n \int_0^\infty \{h(z_i, t, \hat{\beta}) - E_*(t, \hat{\beta})\}dN_i(t).$$

Here,

$$h(z_i, t, \hat{\beta}) = -z_i \ln(1 + e^{\hat{\beta}^T z_i} \hat{\Lambda}_0(t)), \quad E_*(t, \hat{\beta}) = \frac{S_*^{(1)}(t, \hat{\beta})}{S^{(0)}(t, \hat{\beta})}, \quad \text{and}$$

$$S_*^{(1)}(t, \hat{\beta}) = -\sum_{i=1}^n z_i Y_i(t) e^{\hat{\beta}^T z_i} \ln(1 + e^{\hat{\beta}^T z_i} \hat{\Lambda}_0(t)).$$

The statistic U is p-dimensional. The test is based on this modified score statistic and its asymptotic distribution.

Theorem 1: Asymptotic distribution of the modified score statistic
Under some regularity conditions, the statistic

$$T = n^{-1}U^T \hat{D}^{-1} U$$

has an asymptotic χ_p^2 distribution, where p is the dimension of β and $\hat{D} = \hat{\Sigma}_{**}(\tau) - \hat{\Sigma}_*(\tau)\hat{\Sigma}_0^{-1}(\tau)\hat{\Sigma}_*^T(\tau)$ is a consistent estimator of the limit covariance matrix of the random vector $n^{-1/2}U$.

The null hypothesis is rejected with the asymptotic significance level α if $T > \chi_{\alpha,p}^2$; where $\chi_{\alpha,p}^2$ is the α-critical value of the chi-square distribution with p degrees of freedom.

7.4.1 Examples

Example 1. Klein and Moeschberger (2003) analyze the data of death times of elderly residents ($z = 1$, male; $z = 0$, female) of a retirement community.

The number of individuals is 462 (97 males and 365 females). Due to missing values, 458 of 462 observations were used. The data consists of time (in month) when member of the community died or left the center and age when individuals entered the community. The life lengths are left truncated because an individual must survive to a sufficient age to enter the retirement community; all individuals who died earlier and would not enter the center are considered left truncated. The estimate of parameter β is 0.3160.

The value of test statistic T is 1.4399, the p-value is 0.2301. The assumption of PH model is not rejected. The methods described by Kleinbaum and Klein (2005) yield the same results: the plots of logarithm of cumulative hazard function looks reasonably parallel.

Example 2 (continuation of Example 4, Sect. 7.3) This example illustrates the case of left truncated and right-censored data. Suppose that in UIS the subjects are followed-up after they have completed the treatment program, but the drug free period (survival time) is defined as beginning at the time the subject entered the treatment program. In this case, only those subjects who completed the treatment program are included in the analysis, i.e., data are left truncated. Of the 628 subjects, 546 remained drug free for the duration of their treatment program. Due to missing data in covariates, the model is based on 504 of the 546 observations. The estimated coefficients are given in Table 7.2.

The value of test statistic T is 12.1233 ($\sim \chi_{10}^2$), the p-value is 0.2769. The assumption of the Cox model is not rejected.

Table 7.2 The estimated coefficient of covariates

Covariate	Parameter estimate	Standard error	χ^2-value	$Pr > \chi^2$	Hazard ratio
AGE	−0.0332	0.0109	9.2714	0.0023	0.967
becktota	0.0045	0.0053	0.7246	0.3946	1.005
NDRUGFP1	−0.5461	0.1427	14.6401	0.0001	0.579
NDRUGFP2	−0.2038	0.0549	13.7995	0.0002	0.816
IVHX_3	0.2151	0.1185	3.2931	0.0696	1.240
RACE	−0.4945	0.1424	12.0514	0.0005	0.610
TREAT	0.1396	0.1050	1.7664	0.1838	1.150
SITE	−0.9601	0.5559	2.9831	0.0841	0.383
AGEXSITE	0.0398	0.0171	5.4253	0.0198	1.041
RACEXSITE	0.2203	0.2896	0.5788	0.4468	1.246

Table 7.3 The estimated coefficients

Covariate	DF	Parameter estimate	Standard error	Chi-Square	Pr > ChiSq	Hazard ratio
SEX	1	0.15246	0.16234	0.8820	0.3477	1.165
CHF	1	0.88820	0.15921	31.1244	<0.0001	2.431
MI ORDER	1	0.42266	0.16237	6.7759	0.0092	1.526
MITYPE	1	−0.07956	0.16424	0.2346	0.6281	0.924

Example 3. This example also illustrates the case of left truncated and right-censored data. The data given in Hosmer et al (2008) are from The Worcester Heart Attack Study (WHAS). The main goal of this study is to describe the trend over time in the incidence and survival rates following hospital admission for acute myocardial infarction (AMI). The time variable is total length of hospital stay (that is the days between the date of last follow-up and hospital admission date). The censoring variable is the status of last follow-up (0, alive; 1, dead). The left truncation variable is the length of hospital stay between hospital discharge and hospital admission. Subjects who died in the hospital are not included in the analysis. The covariates are sex (0, male; 1, female), left heart failure complications (CHF: 0, no; 1, yes), MI order (MIORD: 0, first; 1, recurrent), MI type (MITYPE: 1, Q-wave; 0, not Q-wave). Due to missing data in covariates, the analysis is based on 392 observations. The estimated coefficients are given in Table 7.3.

The value of the test statistic T is 12.66 ($\sim \chi_4^2$), the p-value is 0.0131. The assumption of the Cox model is rejected. The method based on Schoenfeld residuals (not reported here) yields the same result.

Chapter 8
Remarks on Computations in Parametric and Semiparametric Estimation

The literature on parametric and nonparametric estimation for models considered in the previous chapters is enormous. See, for example, Wu et al. (2002), Dabrowska (2005, 2006), Bagdonavicius and Nikulin (1999, 2002, 2005), Martinussen and Scheike (2006), Scheike (2006), Zeng and Lin (2007), etc. Methods of estimation depend on experimental plans, censoring mechanism, covariate types, etc. Here we only give two general approaches, for parametric and semiparametric cases, which work well for all models. We have several remarks to help clarify the considered models.

Remark 1. Additive hazards model and its generalizations
We know that an alternative of the PH model is the *additive hazards* (AH) model:

$$\lambda_{x(\cdot)}(t) = \lambda_0(t) + \beta^T x(t),$$

where β is the vector of regression parameters. If the AH model holds then the difference of default rates under constant covariates does not depend on t. Like the PH model, this model has the absence of memory property: the default rate at the moment t does not depend on the values of the covariate before the moment t.

Usually the AH model is used in the semiparametric form: the parameters β and the baseline rate λ_0 are both unknown.

We know also that both the PH and AH models are included in the *additive-multiplicative hazards* (AMH) model (Lin and Ying 1996):

$$\lambda_{x(\cdot)}(t) = e^{\beta^T x(t)} \lambda_0(t) + \gamma^T x(t).$$

This model also has the absence of memory property.

A modification of the AH model for constant covariates is the *Aalen's additive risk* (AAR) model (Aalen 1980): the default rate under the covariate x is modeled by a linear combination of several baseline rates with covariate components as coefficients:

© The Author(s) 2016
M. Nikulin and H.-D.I. Wu, *The Cox Model and Its Applications*,
SpringerBriefs in Statistics, DOI 10.1007/978-3-662-49332-8_8

$$\lambda_x(t) = x^T\alpha(t).$$

where $\alpha(t) = (\lambda_1(t), \dots, \lambda_m(t))^T$ is an unknown vector function.

Both AH and AAR models are included in the *partly parametric additive risk* (PPAR) model (McKeague and Sasieni 1994):

$$\lambda_x(t) = x_1^T\alpha(t) + \beta^T x_2,$$

where x_1 and x_2 are q- and p-dimensional components of the explanatory variable x, $\alpha(t) = (\lambda_1(t), \dots, \lambda_q(t))^T$ and $\beta = (\beta_1, \dots, \beta_p)^T$ are unknown.

Analogously, as in the case of the PH model, the AH model can be generalized by the *generalized additive hazards* (GAH) model:

$$\lambda_{x(\cdot)}(t) = q\{\Lambda_{x(\cdot)}(t)\}(\lambda_0(t) + \beta^T x(t)),$$

where the function q is parameterized as in the case of GPH models.

Both the GPH and the GAH models can be included into the *generalized additive-multiplicative hazards* (GAMH) model (Bagdonavicius and Nikulin 1997):

$$\lambda_{x(\cdot)}(t) = q\{\Lambda_{x(\cdot)}(t)\}\left(e^{\beta^T x(t)}\lambda_0(t) + \delta^T x(t)\right).$$

In both GAH and GAMH models the function q is parametrized as in the GPH models: $q(u) = (1+u)^{-\gamma+1}$, $(1+\gamma u)^{-1}$, $e^{-\gamma u}$, and the GAH1, GAH2, GAH3 or GAMH1, GAMH2, GAMH3 models are obtained.

Remark 2. For *parametric* models, the maximum likelihood (ML) estimation procedure gives the best estimators. For simplicity let us consider only the "right-censored" data (which is typical in survival analysis):

$$(X_1, \delta_1, x_1(\cdot)), \dots, (X_n, \delta_n, x_n(\cdot)), \tag{8.1}$$

where $X_i = \min(T_i, C_i)$, $\delta_i = \mathbf{1}_{\{T_i \le C_i\}}$ for $i = 1, \dots, n,$; T_i and C_i are the failure and censoring times, $\mathbf{1}_A$ is the indicator of an event A, and $x_i(\cdot)$ is the covariate corresponding to the ith subject. Equivalently, right-censored data can be presented in the following form:

$$(N_1(t), Y_1(t), x_1(t), t \ge 0), \dots, (N_n(t), Y_n(t), x_n(\cdot), \quad t \ge 0), \tag{8.2}$$

where $N_i(t) = \mathbf{1}_{\{X_i \le t, \delta_i = 1\}}$ is the counting process and $Y_i(t) = \mathbf{1}_{\{X_i \ge t\}}$ is the "at-risk" process for subject i, respectively. Further, for any $t > 0$,

$$N(t) = \sum_{i=1}^{n} N_i(t) \quad \text{and} \quad Y(t) = \sum_{i=1}^{n} Y_i(t)$$

are the number of observed failures in the interval $[0, t]$ and the number of at-risk subjects just prior to time t. The *compensators* of the counting processes N_i with respect to the *history* of the observed processes are $\int Y_i \lambda_i du$.

Remark 3. Suppose that the survival distributions of all n subjects given $x_i(\cdot)$ are *absolutely continuous* with survival functions $S_i(t, \theta)$ and hazard rates $\lambda_i(t, \theta)$, indexed by $\theta \in \Theta \subset \mathbf{R}^s$; and that the distributions of C_i and $x_i(\cdot)$ do not depend on θ. The likelihood function for θ is

$$L(\theta) = \prod_{i=1}^{n} \lambda_i^{\delta_i}(X_i, \theta) \, S_i(X_i, \theta),$$

or,

$$L(\theta) = \prod_{i=1}^{n} \left(\int_0^\infty \lambda_i(u, \theta) \, dN_i(u) \right)^{\delta_i} \exp\left\{ -\int_0^\infty Y_i(u) \lambda_i(u, \theta) \, du \right\}. \quad (8.3)$$

The ML estimator $\hat{\theta}$ of the parameter θ maximizes the likelihood function. It satisfies the equation $U(\hat{\theta}) = 0$, where U is the score function:

$$U(\theta) = \frac{\partial}{\partial \theta} \ln L(\theta) = \sum_{i=1}^{n} \int_0^\infty \frac{\partial}{\partial \theta} \log \lambda_i(u, \theta) \{ dN_i(u) - Y_i(u) \lambda_i(u, \theta) \} du. \quad (8.4)$$

The form of the hazards rates λ_i for the PH, AFT, GPH, AH, AMH, GAH, GAMH is given by the corresponding formulas in Chaps. 3–7. The parameter θ contains the regression parameter β, the complementary parameter γ (for some models), and the baseline hazard λ_0 (which could be taken from some parametric family).

Remark 4. For *semiparametric* estimation, we expose shortly a general approach proposed by Bagdonavičius and Nikulin (1998, 1999, 2002) based on the *modified partial likelihood* when λ_0 is unknown. (See also Dabrowska 2005–2007, Martinussen and Scheike 2006.) The martingale property of the difference

$$N_i(t) - \int_0^t Y_i(u) \lambda_i(u, \theta) du \quad (8.5)$$

implies a "pseudo estimator" (which depends on θ) of the baseline cumulative hazard Λ_0. Indeed, all the above-considered models can be classified into three groups depending on the form of $\lambda_i(t, \theta) dt$. It is of the form

$$g(x_i(s), \ \Lambda_0(s), \ 0 \le s \le t, \ \theta) d\Lambda_0(t)$$

for PH, GPH, CE models, $d\Lambda_0(f_i(t, \theta))$ for AFT, CHSS models, and

$$g_1(x_i(s), \ \Lambda_0(s), \ 0 \le s \le t, \ \theta) d\Lambda_0(t) + g_2(x_i(s), \ \Lambda_0(s), \ 0 \le s \le t, \ \theta) dt$$

for AH, AMH, GAH, GAMH models. Estimation for the PH and AFT models with time-dependent regression coefficients and time-dependent covariates is analogous to the estimation for the PH and AFT models with constant regression coefficients and properly chosen time-dependent covariates.

Remark 5. For the first group of models, the martingale property of the difference (8.5) implies the recurrently defined "estimator":

$$\tilde{\Lambda}_0(t, \theta) = \int_0^t \frac{dN(u)}{\sum_{j=1}^n Y_j(u) g(x_j(v), \tilde{\Lambda}_0(v, \theta), 0 \le v < u, \theta)}.$$

For the second group,

$$\tilde{\Lambda}_0(t, \theta) = \sum_{i=1}^n \int_0^t \frac{dN_i(h_i(u, \theta))}{\sum_{l=1}^n Y_l(h_l(u, \theta))},$$

where $h_i(u, \theta)$ is the function inverse to $f_i(u, \theta)$ with respect to the first argument.

Note that for PH, GPH1, GPH2, GPH3 models,

$$g(x(s), \Lambda_0(s), 0 \le s \le t, \theta) = e^{\beta^T x(t)}, \quad e^{\beta^T x(t)} \left(1 + \gamma \int_0^t e^{\beta^T x(u)} d\Lambda_0(u)\right)^{\frac{1}{\gamma}-1},$$

$$e^{\beta^T x(t)} \left(1 + 2\gamma \int_0^t e^{\beta^T x(u)} d\Lambda_0(u)\right)^{-\frac{1}{2}}, \quad e^{\beta^T x(t)} \left(1 + \gamma \int_0^t e^{\beta^T x(u)} d\Lambda_0(u)\right)^{-1},$$

respectively. For the CE model

$$g(x(s), \Lambda_0(s), 0 \le s \le t, \theta) = e^{\beta^T x(t)} \{1 + \Lambda_{x(\cdot)}(t)\}^{1 - e^{\gamma^T x(t)}},$$

where the function $\Lambda_{x(\cdot)}$ is defined by the equation

$$\int_0^t e^{\beta^T x(u)} \{1 + \Lambda_{x(\cdot)}(u)\}^{1 - e^{\gamma^T x(u)}} d\Lambda_0(u) = \Lambda_{x(\cdot)}(t).$$

If x is constant in time then for the CE model

$$g(x, \Lambda_0(s), 0 \le s \le t, \theta) = e^{\beta^T x} \{1 + e^{(\beta+\gamma)^T x} \Lambda_0(t)\}^{e^{-\gamma^T x} - 1}.$$

Moreover, for the AFT model,

$$f_i(t, \theta) = \int_0^t e^{-\beta^T x(u)} du;$$

and for the AH, AMH, GAH, and GAMH models,

$$g_1(x_i(s), \Lambda_0(s), 0 \le s \le t, \theta) = 1, \quad e^{\beta^T x(t)}, \quad x^T, \quad x_1^T$$

and

$$g_2(x_i(s), \Lambda_0(s), 0 \le s \le t, \theta) = \beta^T x(t), \quad \beta^T x(t), \quad 0, \quad \beta_2^T x(t),$$

respectively.

Remark 6. For the GAMH1 model:

$$g_1(x_i(s), \Lambda_0(s), 0 \le s \le t, \theta) = e^{\beta^T x(t)} g(x_i(s), \Lambda_0(s), 0 \le s \le t, \theta),$$
$$g_2(x_i(s), \Lambda_0(s), 0 \le s \le t, \theta) = \delta^T x(t) g(x_i(s), \Lambda_0(s), 0 \le s \le t, \theta),$$

where

$$g(x_i(s), \Lambda_0(s), 0 \le s \le t, \theta) = \left(1 + \gamma \left(\int_0^t e^{\beta^T x(u)} d\Lambda_0(u) + \delta^T \int_0^t x(u) du\right)\right)^{\frac{1}{\gamma} - 1}.$$

Analogous formulas for the GAMH2, GAMH3, GAH1, GAH2, and GAH3 models can be expressed in a similar manner.

For the PH, GPH, and CE models the weight $\frac{\partial}{\partial \theta} \log \lambda_i(u, \theta)$ in (8.4) is a function of $x_i(\cdot)(v), \Lambda_0(v), 0 \le v \le u$ and θ. So the modified score function is obtained from replacing Λ_0 by a consistent estimator $\tilde{\Lambda}_0$ in the parametric score function (8.4).

In the case of the AFT, AH, AMH models, the weight depends not only on Λ_0 but also on λ_0 and/or λ_0'. Here $\lambda_i(u)du$ does not depend on λ_0 and λ_0'. The construction of the modified likelihood function can be done by different ways. For example, one can replace Λ_0 by $\tilde{\Lambda}_0$, λ_0 and λ_0' by their nonparametric kernel estimators which are easily obtained from the estimator $\tilde{\Lambda}_0$.

Remark 7. Computation of the modified likelihood estimators is simple for the PH, GPH, and CE models. It is due to the remarkable fact that these estimators can be obtained by the partial likelihood function expressed as:

$$L_P(\theta) = \prod_{i=1}^n \left[\int_0^\infty \frac{g\{x_i(v), \Lambda_0(v), 0 \le v \le u, \theta\}}{\sum_{j=1}^n Y_j(u) g\{x_j(v), \Lambda_0(v), 0 \le v \le u, \theta\}} dN_i(u) \right]^{\delta_i}, \quad (8.6)$$

and suppose at first that Λ_0 is known. If Λ_0 in the score function is substituted by $\tilde{\Lambda}_0$, then exactly the same modified score function is obtained as if it has come from the full likelihood.

In conclusion, it is better to maximize the modified partial likelihood function, which is simply the partial likelihood function (8.6) except for replacing Λ_0 by $\tilde{\Lambda}_0$. The general quasi-Newton optimization algorithm (such as that given in R language) works well for seeking the maximizer of θ. Note that the modified maximum likelihood estimators are the values of θ minimizing the distance of the modified score function from zero. Computational methods for such estimators are also given in Lin and Geyer (1992), Hsieh (2001), Wu et al. (2002), Wu (2007), Dabrowska (2005, 2006), Martinussen and Scheike (2006).

Remark 8. PH model with time-dependent regression coefficients

Flexible models can be obtained by supposing that the regression coefficients β in the PH model are time-dependent (see Sect. 5.3):

$$\lambda_{x(\cdot)}(t) = e^{\beta(t)^T x(t)} \lambda_0(t), \tag{8.7}$$

where

$$\beta^T(t)\,x(t) = \sum_{i=1}^{m} \beta_i(t) x_i(t).$$

If the function $\beta_i(\cdot)$ is increasing or decreasing in time then the effect of the ith component of the explanatory variable is increasing or decreasing.

Usually the coefficients $\beta_i(t)$ are considered in the form

$$\beta_i(t) = \beta_i + \gamma_i g_i(t), \quad (i = 1, 2, \ldots, m),$$

where $g_i(t)$ are some *specified* functions such as t, $\ln t$, $\ln(1 + t)$, $(1 + t)^{-1}$, or realizations of predictable processes. In such a case the PH model with time-dependent coefficients can be written in the usual form where the "covariables" contain $x_i(\cdot)$ and $x_i(\cdot)g_i(\cdot)$. Specifically, let

$$\theta = (\theta_1, \ldots, \theta_{2m})^T = (\beta_1, \ldots, \beta_m, \gamma_1, \ldots, \gamma_m)^T,$$
$$z(\cdot) = (z_1(\cdot), \ldots, z_{2m}(\cdot))^T = (x_1(\cdot), \ldots, x_m(\cdot), x_1(\cdot)g_1(\cdot), \ldots, x_m(\cdot)g_m(\cdot))^T,$$

then

$$\beta^T(u)x(u) = \sum_{i=1}^{m}(\beta_i + \gamma_i g_i(t))\,x_i(t) = \theta^T z(u).$$

So the PH model with time-dependent regression coefficients can be written as

$$\lambda_{x(\cdot)}(t) = e^{\theta^T z(t)} \lambda_0(t).$$

We have the PH model with time-dependent "covariables" and constant "regression parameters." Methods of estimation for the usual PH model are still applicable. Note that the introduced "covariables" have time-dependent components even in the case when the covariable x is constant over time.

An alternative method is to take $\beta_i(t)$ as piecewise constant functions with jumps as unknown parameters. In this case the PH model is used locally and the ratios of the default rates under constant covariates are constant at each time interval.

Chapter 9
Cox Model for Degradation and Failure Time Data

9.1 Aging and Longevity, Failure and Degradation

It is well known that traditionally the failure time data are used for product reliability estimation or for estimation of survival characteristics. Failures of highly reliable units are *rare* and other information should be used in addition to censored failure time data. *One way* of obtaining a complementary reliability information is to use higher levels of experimental factors or covariates (such as temperature, voltage, or pressure) to increase the number of failures and, hence, to obtain reliability information quickly. The *accelerated life testing* (ALT) of biotechnical systems is a simple practical method for estimation of reliability of new systems without having to wait for the operating lives of them. It is evident that the *extrapolating reliability* from ALT always carries the risk that the accelerating stresses do not properly excite the failure mechanism which dominates at operating (*normal*) stresses.

Another way of obtaining this complementary survival information is to measure some parameters (covariates) which characterize the aging of the system in time. In *longevity* analysis of highly reliable complex industrial or biological systems, the degradation processes provide additional information about the *aging, degradation,* and *deterioration* of systems. From this point of view the *degradation data* are rich sources of reliability information and have *advantages* over failure time data. Degradation is *natural response* for some tests. With degradation data it is possible to make useful reliability and statistical inference, even with no failures. Sometimes it is possible to construct the *expert's estimation* of the level of degradation.

Degradation Process

In reliability considerable interests lies in constructing a *covariates process* $Z(\cdot) = Z_r(\cdot)$ which describes the *real* process of *wear, fatigue,* or the *usage history* up to time t. Note that he history indicates the level of fatigue, degradation, and deterioration of a system and may influence on the rate of degradation, the risk of

© The Author(s) 2016
M. Nikulin and H.-D.I. Wu, *The Cox Model and Its Applications*,
SpringerBriefs in Statistics, DOI 10.1007/978-3-662-49332-8_9

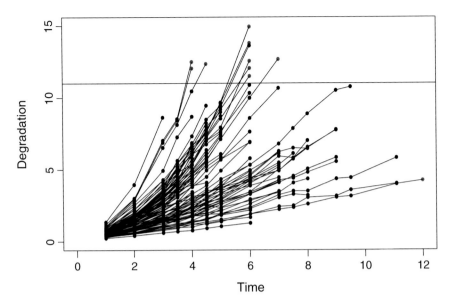

Fig. 9.1 Fatigue Crack Size for Alloy-A and Nonlinear fitting of Paris curves with nls and gnl

failure and the reliability of system. Statistical modeling of *observed degradation* processes can help understand different real physical, chemical, medical, biological, physiological, social or economic degradation processes of aging (Fig. 9.1).

Information about *real degradation* processes help us to construct the degradation models with which the *cumulative damage* can be predicted. By the main idea of degradation models a *soft failure* is observed if the degradation process reaches a *critical threshold* z_0. A soft failure caused by degradation occurs when $Z_r(t)$ reaches the value z_0. The *moment* $T^{(0)}$ of *soft failure* is defined by

$$T^{(0)} = \sup\{t : Z_r(t) < z_0\} = \inf\{t : Z_r(t) \geq z_0\}.$$

So it is reasonable to construct the so-called *degradation models*, based on some suppositions about the mathematical properties of the degradation process $Z_r(\cdot)$, according to the observed *longitudinal* data in the experiment. It is evident that both considered methods may be combined to construct the so-called *joint degradation* models. For this it is enough to define a failure of system when its degradation (*internal wear*) reaches a critical value or a *traumatic event* (failure) occurs. The joint degradation models form the class of models with *competing risk*, since for any item we consider two competing causes of failure: degradation, reaching a *threshold* (soft failure), and occurrence of a *hard* or *traumatic failure*. Let T be the moment of *traumatic failure* of a unit. In considered class of models the *failure time* τ is the *minimum* of the moments of traumatic and soft failures,

$$\tau = \min(T^{(0)}, T) = T^{(0)} \wedge T.$$

These models are also called *degradation-threshold-shock models*. For such models the degradation process $Z_r(t)$ can be considered as an additional time varying covariate, which describes the *process of wear* or the *usage history up to time t*.

The *convex and concave degradation models* are interesting to use to study the growth of tumors. To model the degradation-failure time process, Meeker and Escobar (1998) and Lawless (2003) used *general degradation path models*, according to which

$$Z_r(t) = g(t, A).$$

Here $A = (A_1, \ldots, A_l)$ is a random vector with positive components and g is a specified continuously differentiable function of t, which increases from 0 to $+\infty$ with t. For example, if $l = 1$, we have $A = A_1$—a positive random variable; and if

$$g(t, A) = t/A, \quad A \in R_+^1,$$

we have a *linear degradation*. If $l = 2$ and

$$g(t, A) = (t/A_1)^{A_2},$$

we have a *convex* or *concave* degradation. It is also assumed that, for each $t > 0$, the *degradation path*

$$g(s, a), \quad 0 < s \le t,$$

determines in the *unique way* the value a of the random vector A. For another example we consider

$$Z_r(t) = \int_0^t e^{W(s)} ds$$

where $W(\cdot)$ is a random process (say, a *Wiener process*) with continuous trajectories.

Degradation is modeled by the process $Z(t, A)$, where t is time and A is some possibly multidimensional random variable. Nelson (1990) and Meeker and Escobar (1998) introduced *linear degradation models* to study the increase in a resistance measurement over time, and the *convex and concave degradation models* to study the *growth of tumors*. *Concave degradation models* may also be used to describe degradation of components in electronic circuits in medical equipments. Moreover, Lawless (2003), Meeker and Escobar (1998), Kahle and Wendt (2006), Lehmann (2004), Bagdonavicius and Nikulin (2002) described many different applications and models for *accelerated degradation* with data involving destructive testings.

Influence of covariates on degradation is also modeled in Meeker and Escobar (1998), Bagdonavicius and Nikulin (2001, 2002, 2004, 2006), Nikulin et al. (2010) to estimate survival when the *environment is dynamic*.

In practice the real degradation process $Z_r(t)$ often is *not observed*, and we have to estimate it. In this case we have to work with the *observed degradation process*

$Z(t)$ different from the real degradation process $Z_r(t)$. We suppose that the observed degradation process

$$Z(t) = Z_r(t)U(t), \quad t > 0,$$

where

$$\ln U(t) = V(t) = \sigma W(c(t)),$$

W is the standard *Wiener process* independent of A, and c is a specified continuous increasing function, with $c(0) = 0$.

For any $t > 0$ the *median* of $U(t)$ is 1. This setting permits us to construct a *degradation model with a noise*.

9.2 Joint Model

An important class of models based on degradation processes was developed recently by Wulfsohn and Tsiatis (1997) and Bagdonavičius et al. (2005). Wulfsohn and Tsiatis considered the so-called *joint model* for *survival and longitudinal* data measured with *error*, given by

$$\lambda_T(t|A) = \lambda_0(t)e^{\beta(A_1+A_2t)}, \quad t > 0, \quad (l = 2),$$

where $A = (A_1, A_2)$ follows bivariate normal distribution. On the other hand, Bagdonavičius and Nikulin (2001, 2002, 2006) proposed the model in terms of conditional survival function of T given the *real degradation process*:

$$S_T(t|A) = P\{T > t|g(s, A), 0 \le s \le t\}$$
$$= \exp\left\{-\int_0^t \lambda_0(s, \theta)\lambda(g(s, A))ds\right\},$$

where λ is the *unknown intensity function* and $\lambda_0(s, \theta)$ is the hazard function from a *parametric* family. The distribution of A is not *specified*.

This model states that the conditional hazard rate $\lambda_T(t|A)$ at the moment t given the degradation $g(s, A), 0 \le s \le t$, has the *multiplicative form* as in the *Cox model*:

$$\lambda_T(t|A) = \lambda_0(t, \theta)\lambda(g(t, A)).$$

If

$$\lambda_0(t, \theta) = (1 + t)^\theta \quad \text{or} \quad \lambda_0(t, \theta) = e^{t\theta},$$

then $\theta = 0$ corresponds to the case when the hazard rate at any moment t is a function of *degradation level* at this moment. One can note that in the second model the function λ, which characterizes the *influence* of degradation on the hazard rate, is *nonparametric*; whereas in the Wulfsohn and Tsiatis model this function is *parametric*.

The degradation models with covariates are well adapted for statistical analysis of survival or failure data in *dynamic environments*, and for models the intensity of traumatic failure is an increasing function of degradation level. It is a powerful tool that allows us to *identify precisely the mechanisms that could cause problems at operating stresses*. The *degradation model with covariate* is given by $Z_{x(\cdot)}(t)$. It is used to estimate reliability when the environment is dynamic. The *moment of soft failure* caused by the *degradation* under the covariate $x(\cdot)$ is defined as

$$T_{x(\cdot)}^{(0)} = \sup\{t : Z_{x(\cdot)}(t) < z_0\}.$$

Often the covariates cannot be controlled by an experimenter in such a case. For example, the tire wear rate depends on the quality of roads, temperature, and other factors. Optimization problem for the covariate value was considered by Ceci and Mazliak (2004).

Levy process is a common degradation processes. As an example, consider a *gamma process* with a change of scale (similar to one of the *AFT* model):

$$Z_{x(\cdot)}(t) = \sigma^2 \gamma \left(\int_0^t e^{\beta^T x(s)} ds \right), \quad x(\cdot) \in E.$$

Traumatic event occurs as a stochastic *Poisson process* with a *killing rate* $\lambda\big(Z_{x(\cdot)}(t), x(t)\big)$. Here $\gamma(t)$ is a process with *independent increments* such that

$$\gamma(t) \sim G(1, \nu(t)) = G\left(1, \frac{m(t)}{\sigma^2}\right).$$

That is, for any fixed $t > 0$, the random variable $\gamma(t)$ has the *gamma distribution* with *scale* parameter 1 and the *shape* $\nu(t) = m(t)/\sigma^2$. The density of $\gamma(t)$ is

$$f_{\gamma(t)}(x) = \frac{x^{\nu(t)-1}}{\Gamma(\nu(t))} e^{-x}, \quad x > 0.$$

In this case $\mathbf{E}\gamma(t) = m(t)$ and $\mathbf{Var}\gamma(t) = \sigma^2 m(t)$.

The following four cases are remarkable:

(a) when $\lambda(z, x) = \lambda_0$, the intensity *does not* depend on the degradation and covariates;

(b) when $\lambda(z, x) = e^{\beta^T x}$, the intensity depends only on *covariates* via the *PH* setting;

(c) when $\lambda(z, x) = \lambda_0 + \lambda_1 z$, the intensity depends *linearly* on degradation only;
(d) when $\lambda(z, x) = e^{\beta^T x}(1 + \lambda_1 z)$, the intensity depends *linearly* on degradation and *exponentially* on covariates.

The *semiparametric analysis* of several new degradation and failure time regression models given in terms of $\lambda(x(t), Z_{x(\cdot)}(t))$, with or without covariables, is described in Bagdonavicus and Nikulin (2006).

References

Aalen, O. (1980). A model for nonparametric regression analysis of counting processes. In W. Klonecki, A. Kozek, & J. Rosinski (Eds.), *Mathematical statistics and probability theory* (Vol. 2, pp. 1–25). Lecture notes in statistics. New York: Springer.

Aalen, O. (1988). Heterogeneity in survival analysis. *Statistics in Medicine, 7,* 1121–1137.

Aalen, O. (1992). Modelling heterogeneity in survival analysis by the compound Poisson distribution. *The Annals of Applied Probability, 2,* 951–972.

Aalen, O. (1994). Effects of frailty in survival analysis. *Statistical Methods in Medical Research, 3,* 227–243.

Andersen, P. K., Borgan, O., Gill, R., & Keiding, N. (1993). *Statistical models based on counting processes.* New York: Springer.

Andersen, P. K., & Gill, R. D. (1982). Cox's regression model for counting processes: A large sample study. *The Annals of Statistics, 10,* 1100–1120.

Aven, T., & Jensen, U. (1999). *Stochastic models in reliability.* New York: Springer.

Bagdonavičius, V. (1978). Testing the hyphothesis of the additive accumulation of damages. *Probability Theory and its Applications, 23*(2), 403–408.

Bagdonavičius, V., & Nikulin, M. (1994). Stochastic models of accelerated life. In J. Gutierrez & M. Valderrama (Eds.), *Advanced topics in stochastic modelling* (pp. 73–87). Singapore: World Scientific.

Bagdonavičius, V., & Nikulin, M. (1995). *Semiparametric models in accelerated life testing* (Vol. 98, 70 p). Queen's papers in pure and applied mathematics. Kingston, Canada: Queen's University.

Bagdonavicius, V., & Nikulin, M. (1997a). Transfer functionals and semiparametric regression models. *Biometrika, 84*(2), 365–378.

Bagdonavicius, V., & Nikulin, M. (1997b). Asymptotical analysis of semiparametric models in survival analysis and accelerated life testing. *Statistics, 29*(3), 261–284.

Bagdonavičius, V., & Nikulin, M. (1998a). *Additive and multiplicative semiparametric models in accelerated life testing and survival analysis* (Vol. 108, 109 p). Queen's papers in pure and applied mathematics. Kingston: Queen's university.

Bagdonavicius, V., & Nikulin, M. (1998b). On semiparametric estimation of reliability from accelerated life data. In N. Limnios & D. Ionescu (Eds.), *Mathematical methods in reliability* (pp. 75–89). Boston: Birkhauser.

Bagdonavicius, V., & Nikulin, M. (1999). Generalized proportional hazards model based on modified partial likelihood. *Lifetime Data Analysis, 5,* 323–344.

Bagdonavicius, V., & Nikulin, M. (2000a). On goodness of fit for the linear transformation and frailty models. *Statistics and Probability Letters, 47*(2), 177–188.

Bagdonavicius, V., & Nikulin, M. (2000b). On nonparametric estimation in accelerated experiments with step stresses. *Statistics, 31*(4), 349–365.

© The Author(s) 2016

M. Nikulin and H.-D.I. Wu, *The Cox Model and Its Applications,*
SpringerBriefs in Statistics, DOI 10.1007/978-3-662-49332-8

Bagdonavicius, V., & Nikulin, M. (2001a). Goodness-of-fit tests for the generalized risk models. In N. Balakrishnan, I. A. Ibragimov, & V. N. Nevzorov (Eds.), *Asymptotic methods in probability and statistics with applications* (pp. 385–394). Boston: Birkhauser.

Bagdonavicius, V., & Nikulin, M. (2001b). Mathematical models in the theory of accelerated experiments. In A. A. Ashor & A.-S. F. Obada (Eds.), *Mathematics and the 21st century* (pp. 271–303). Singapore: World Scientific.

Bagdonavicius, V., & Nikulin, M. (2001c). On goodness-of-fit for accelerated life models. *Comptes Rendus, Academie des Sciences de Paris, 332*(1), 171–176. Série I.

Bagdonavičius, V., & Nikulin, M. (2002a). *Accelerated life models*. Boca Raton: Chapman&Hall/CRC.

Bagdonavičius, V., Hafdi, M., El Himdi, K., & Nikulin, M. (2002b). Statistical analysis of the generalised linear proportionnal hazards model, *Proceedings of the Steklov Mathematical Institute, St. Petersburg: Probability and Statistics* (Vol. 6, pp. 5–18). (ISSN 0373-2703).

Bagdonavicius, V., Gerville-Réache, L., & Nikulin, M. (2002c). On parametric inference for step-stresses models. *IEEE Transaction on Reliability, 1*, 27–31.

Bagdonavicius, V., & Nikulin, M. (2002d). Goodness-of-fit tests for accelerated life models. In C. Huber, N. Balakrishnan, M. Nikulin, & M. Mesbah (Eds.), *Goodness-of-fit tests and model validity* (pp. 281–300). Boston: Birkhauser.

Bagdonavicus, V., Cheminade, O., & Nikulin, M. (2004a). Statistical planning and inference in accelerated life testing using the CHSS model. *Journal of the Statistical Planning and Inference, 2*, 535–551.

Bagdonavičius, V., Hafdi, M., & Nikulin, M. (2004b). Analysis of survival data with cross-effects of survival functions. *Biostatistics, 5*(3), 415–425.

Bagdonavičius, V., Levuliene, R., Nikulin, M., & Cheminade, O. (2004c). Tests for the equality of survival distributions against non-location alternatives. *Lifetime Data Analysis, 10*(4), 445–460.

Bagdonavičius, V., & Nikulin, M. (2005). Analyse of survival data with non-proportional hazards and crossing of survival functions. In L. Edler & C. Kitsos (Eds.), *Quantitative methods in cancer and human health risk assessment* (pp. 197–209). New York: Wiley.

Bagdonavičius, V., Haghighi, F., & Nikulin, M. (2005). Statistical analysis of general degradation path model and failure time data with multiple failure modes. *Communication in Statistics. Theory and Methods, 34*(8), 1771–1772.

Bagdonavičius, V., & Nikulin, M. (2006). On goodness-of-fit for homogeneity and proportional hazards. *Applied Stochastic Models in Business and Industry, 22*, 607–619.

Bagdonavičius, V., Levuliene, R., & Nikulin, M. (2011a). Asymptotic analysis of a new dynamic semiparametric regression models with cross-effects of survival. *Journal of Mathematical Sciences, 176*(2), 117–123.

Bagdonavičius, V., Kruopis, J., & Nikulin, M. (2011b). *Non-parametric tests for censored data (233 p)*. London: ISTE-Wiley.

Bagdonavičius, V., & Nikulin, M. (2011). Chi-squared goodness-of-fit test for righr censored data. *The International Journal of Applied Mathematics and Statistics, 24*, 30–50.

Bednarski, T. (1993). Robust estimation in Cox's regression model. *Scandinavian Journal of Statistics, 20*, 213–225.

Bennett, N. (1983). Log-logistic regression models for survival data. *Applied Statistics, 32*, 165–171.

Bhattacharyya, G. K., & Stoejoeti, Z. (1989). A tampered failure rate model for step-stress accelerated life test. *Communications in Statistics - Theory and Methods, 18*, 1627–1643.

Birnbaum, Z. M., & Saunders, S. C. (1969). A new family of life distributions. *Journal of Applied Probability, 6*, 319–327.

Breslow, N. E. (1974). Covariance analysis of censored survival data. *Biometrics, 30*, 579–594.

Breslow, N. E., Edler, L., & Berger, J. (1984). A two-sample censored-data rank test for acceleration. *Biometrics, 40*, 1049–1062.

Cai, Z., & Sun, Y. (2003). Local linear estimation for time-dependent coefficients in Cox's regression models. *Scandinavian Journal of Statistics, 30*, 93–112.

Ceci, C., & Mazliak, L. (2004). Optimal design in nonparametric life testing. *Statistical Inference for Stochastical Processes*, *7*, 305–325.

Chen, K., Jin, Z., & Ying, Z. (2002). Semiparametric analysis of transformation models with censored data. *Biometrika*, *89*, 659–668.

Cox, D. R. (1972). Regression models and life tables. *Journal of the Royal Statistical Society*, *B34*, 187–220.

Cox, D. R. (1975). Partial likelihood. *Biometrika*, *62*, 269–276.

Cox, D. R., & Oakes, D. (1984). *Analysis of survival data*. London: Chapman and Hall.

Dabrowska, D. (2005). Quantile regression in transformation models. *Sankhya*, *67*, 153–187.

Dabrowska, D. (2006). Estimation in a class of semi-parametric trasformation models. In J. Rojo (Ed.), *Second Eric L. Lehmann symposium - optimality* (Vol. 49, pp. 131–169). Lecture notes and monograph series. Cambridge: Institute of Mathematical Statistics.

Dabrowska, D. (2007). Information bounds and efficient estimation in a class of censored transformation models. *Acta Applicandae Mathematicae*, *96*, 177–201.

Dabrowska, D. M., & Doksum, K. A. (1988). Partial likelihood in transformation model with censored data. *Scandinavian Journal of Statistics*, *15*, 1–23.

Desmond, A. F. (1986). On the relation between two fatigue-life models. *IEEE Transactions on Reliability*, *R–35*, 167–169.

El Fassi, K., Abdous, B., & Mesbah, M. (2009). Ajustement polynomial local de la fonction d'égalisation équipercentil : convergence uniforme presque sûre. *Comptes Rendus de l'Academie des Science*, *347*, 195–200. Serie 1.

Fleming, T. R., O'Fallon, J. R., & O'Brien, P. C. (1980). Modified Kolmogorov-Smirnov test procedures with application to arbitrarily right-censored data. *Biometrics*, *36*, 607–625.

Fleming, T. R., & Harrington, D. P. (1991). *Counting processes and survival analysis*. New York: Wiley.

Gill, R. (1980). *Censoring and stochastic integrals* (Vol. 124). CWI tracts. Amsterdam: Center for Mathematics and Computer Sciences.

Gill, R. D., & Schumacher, M. (1987). A simple test of the proportional hazards assumption. *Biometrika*, *74*, 289–300.

Greenwood, P. E., & Nikulin, M. S. (1996). *A guide to chi-squared testing*. New York: Wiley.

Harrington, D. P., & Fleming, T. R. (1982). A class of rank test procedures for censored survival data. *Biometrika*, *69*, 553–566.

Heritier, S., Cantoni, E., Copt, S., & Victoria-Feser, M. P. (2009). *Robust methods in biostatistics*. New York: Wiley.

Hjort, N. L. (1992). On inference in parametric survival data. *International Statistical Review*, *60*(3), 355–387.

Hosmer, D. W., Lemeshow, S., & May, S. (2008). *Applied survival analysis: Regression modeling of time to event data*. New York: Wiley.

Hougaard, P. (1984). Life table method for heterogeneous populations: distributions describing the heterogeneity. *Biometrika*, *71*, 75–83.

Hougaard, P. (1986). Survival models for heterogeneous populations derived from stable distributions. *Biometrika*, *73*, 387–396.

Hougaard, P. (2000). *Analysis of multivariate survival data*. New York: Springer.

Hsieh, F. (1995). The empirical process approach for semiparametric two-sample models with heterogeneous treatment effect. *Journal of the Royal Statistical Society*, *B57*, 735–748.

Hsieh, F. (1996). A transformation model for two survival curves: An empirical process approach. *Biometrika*, *83*, 519–528.

Hsieh, F. (2001). On heteroscedastic hazards regression models: Theory and application. *Journal of the Royal Statistical Society*, *B63*, 63–79.

Huber-Carol, C., & Nikulin, M. (2008). Extended Cox and accelerated models in reliability, with general censoring and truncation. In F. Vonta, M. Nikulin, N. Limnios, & C. Huber (Eds.), *Statistical models and methods for biomedical and technical systems* (pp. 3–22). Boston: Birkhauser.

Huber-Carol, C., Solev, V., & Vonta, F. (2006). Estimation of density for arbitrarily censored and truncated data. In M. Nikulin, D. Commenges, & C. Huber (Eds.), *Probability, statistics and modelling in public health* (pp. 246–265). New York: Springer.

Johansen, S. (1983). An extension of Coxs regression model. *International Statistical Review, 51,* 165–174.

Kahle, W., & Wendt, H. (2006). Statistical analysis of some parametric degradation models. In M. Nikulin, D. Commenges, & C. Huber (Eds.), *Probability, statistics and modelling in public health* (pp. 266–279). New York: Springer.

Kalbfleisch, J. D., & Prentice, R. L. (2002). *The statistical analysis of failure time data* (2nd ed.). New York: Wiley.

Karnofsky, D. A., & Burchenal, J. M. (1949). The clinical evaluation of chemotherapeutic agents in cancer. In C. M. Macleod (Ed.), *Evaluation of chemotherapeutic agents* (p. 149). New York: Columbia University Press.

Kleinbaum, D. G., & Klein, M. (2005). *Survival analysis: A self-learning text* (2nd ed.). New York: Springer.

Klein, J. P., & Moeschberger, M. L. (2003). *Survival analysis* (2nd ed.). New York: Springer.

Kolen, M. J., & Brennan, R. L. (2004). *Test equating, scaling, and linking methods and practices.* New York: Springer.

Kong, F. H., & Slud, E. (1997). Robust covariate-adjusted logrank tests. *Biometrika, 84,* 847–862.

Kosorok, M., Lee, B. L., & Fine, J. P. (2004). Robust inference for univariate proportional hazards frailty regression models. *Annals of Statistics, 32*(4), 1418–1491.

Koziol, J. A. (1978). A two sample Cramer-von Mises test for randomly censored data. *Biometrical Journal, 20,* 603–608.

Lawless, J. F. (2003). *Statistical models and methods for lifetime data.* New York: Wiley.

Lehmann, A. (2004). On a degradation-failure models for repairable items. In M. Nikulin, N. Balakrishnan, M. Mesbah, & N. Limnios (Eds.), *Parametric and semiparametric models with applications to reliability, survival analysis, and quality of life* (pp. 65–80). Boston: Birkhauser.

Liang, K. Y., Self, S. G., & Liu, X. (1990). The Cox proportional hazards model with change-point : An epidemiologic application. *Biometrics, 46,* 783–793.

Lin, D. Y. (1991). Goodness-of-fit analysis for the Cox regression model based on a class of parameter estimators. *Journal of the American Statistical Association, 86,* 725–728.

Lin, D. Y., & Geyer, C. J. (1992). Computation methods for semiparametric linear regression with censored data. *Journal of Computational and Graphical Statistics, 1,* 77–90.

Lin, C. L., Lin, P. H., Chou, L. W., Lan, S. J., Meng, N. H., Lo, S. F., et al. (2009). Model-based prediction of length of stay for rehabilitating stroke patients. *Journal of the Formosan Medical Association, 108,* 653–662.

Lin, D. Y., & Wei, L. J. (1989). The robust inference for the Cox proportional hazards model. *Journal of the American Statistical Association, 84,* 1074–1078.

Lin, D. Y., & Ying, Z. (1994). Semiparametric analysis of the additive risk model. *Biometrika, 81*(1), 61–71.

Lin, D. Y., & Ying, Z. (1996). Semiparametric analysis of the general additive-multiplicative hazard models for counting processes. *Annals of Statistics, 23*(5), 1712–1734.

Mann, N. R., Schafer, R. E., & Singpurwalla, N. D. (1974). *Methods for statistical analysiss of reliability and lifetime data.* New York: Wiley.

Mantel, N. (1966). Evaluation of survival data and two new rank order statistics arising in its consideration. *Cancer Chemotherapy Report, 50,* 163–170.

Martinussen, T., & Scheike, T. (2006). *Dynamic regression models for survival functions.* New York: Springer.

Marubini, R., & Valsecchi, M. G. (1995). *Analysing survival data from clinical trials and observational studies.* Chichester: Wiley.

Marzec, L., & Marzec, P. (1997). Generalized martingale-residual processes for goodness-of-fit inference in Cox's type regression models. *Annals of Statistics, 25,* 683–714.

McKeague, I. W., & Sasieni, P. D. (1994). A partly parametric additive risk model. *Biometrika*, *81*(3), 501–514.

Meeker, W. Q., & Escobar, L. (1998). *Statistical methods for reliability data*. New York: Wiley.

Miller, R., & Halpern, J. (1982). Regression with censored data. *Biometrika, 59*(3), 521–531.

Minder, C. E., & Bednarski, T. (1996). A robust method for proportional hazards regression. *Statistics in Medicine, 15*, 1033–1047.

Moreau, T., Maccario, J., Lelouch, J., & Huber, C. (1992). Weighted logrank statistics for comparing two distributions. *Biometrika, 79*(14), 195–198.

Mudholkar, G., Srivastava, D., & Freimer, M. (1995). The exponentiated Weibull family: A reanalysis of the bus-motor-failure data. *Technometrics, 37*(14), 436–445.

Mudholkar, G., & Srivastava, D. (1993). Exponentiated Weibull family for analyzing bathtub failure-rate data. *IEEE Transactions on Reliability, 42*(2), 299–302.

Murphy, S. A. (1993). Testing for a time dependent coefficient in Cox's regression model. *Scandinavian Journal of Statistics, 20*, 35–40.

Murphy, S. A., & Sen, P. K. (1991). Time-dependent coefficient in a Cox-type regression model. *Stochastic Processes and Their Applications, 39*, 153–180.

Murphy, S. A., Rossini, A. J., & Van der Vaart, A. W. (1997). Maximum likelihood estimation in the proportional odds model. *Journal of the American Statistical Association, 92*, 968–976.

Nelson, W. (1990). *Accelerated testing*. New York: Wiley.

Nikulin, M. S., Limnios, N., Kahle, W., & Huber-Carol, C. (Eds.). (2010). *Advances in degradation modeling: Applications to reliability, survival analysis, and finance*. Boston: Birkhauser.

Nikulin, M., & Wu, H. (2006). Flexible regression models for carcinogenesis studies. In I. Ibragimov & V. Sudakov (Eds.), *Probability and statistics* (Vol. 10, pp. 78–101). St. Petetsburg: V. Steklov Mathematical Institute.

O'Quigley, J., & Pessione, F. (1991). The problem of a covariate-time qualitative interaction in a survival study. *Biometrics, 47*, 101–115.

Peto, R. (1972). Rank tests of maximal power against Lehmann-type alternatives. *Biometrika, 59*, 472–475.

Peto, R., & Peto, J. (1972). Asymptotically efficient rank invariant test procedures. *Journal of the Royal Statistical Society, A135*, 185–206.

Piantadosi, S. (1997). *Clinical trials*. New York: Wiley.

Quantin, C., Moreau, T., Asselain, B., Maccario, J., & Lellouch, J. (1996). A regression survival model for testing the proportional hazards hypothesis. *Biometrics, 52*, 874–885.

Reid, N., & Crépeau, H. (1985). Influence functions for proportional hazards regression. *Biometrika, 72*, 1–9.

Scheike, T. H. (2006). A flexible semiparametric transformation model for survival data. *Lifetime Data Analysis, 12*, 461–480.

Schoenfeld, D. (1980). Chi-squared goodness-of-fit tests for the proportional hazards regression model. *Biometrika, 67*(145–153), 263–281.

Shaked, M., & Singpurwalla, N. D. (1983). Inference for step-stress accelerated life tests. *Journal of Statistical Planning and Inference, 7*, 295–306.

Sedyakin, N. M. (1966). On one physical principle in reliability theory. *Technical Cybernetics, 3*, 80–87.

Singpurwalla, N. D. (1995). Survival in dynamic environments. *Statistical Science, 1*(10), 86–103.

Solev, V. (2009). Estimation of density on censored data. In M. Nikulin, N. Limnios, N. Balakrishnan, C. Huber, & W. Kahle (Eds.), *Advances in degradation models. Applications to industry, medicine and finance* (pp. 369–380). Boston: Birkhauser.

Stablein, D. M., & Koutrouvelis, I. A. (1985). A two sample test sensitive to crossing hazards in uncensored and singly censored data. *Biometrics, 41*, 643–652.

Tabatabai, M. A., Bursac, Z., Williams, D. K., & Singh, K. P. (2007). Hypertabastic survival model. *Theoretical Biology and Medical Modelling, 4*, 1–13.

Tarone, R. E., & Ware, J. H. (1977). On distribution-free tests for equality for survival distributions. *Biometrika., 64*, 156–160.

Therneau, T. M., & Grambsch, P. M. (2000). *Modeling survival data*. New York: Springer.

Tian, L., Zucker, D., & Wei, L. (2005). On the Cox model with time-varying regression coefficients. *Journal of the American Statistical Association, 100*, 172–183.

Tsiatis, A. A. (1981). A large sample study of Cox's regression model. *Annals of Statistics, 9*, 93–108.

Tubert-Bitter, P., Kramar, A., Chalé, J. J., & Moreau, T. (1994). Linear rank tests for comparing survival in two groups with crossing hazards. *Computational Statistics and Data Analysis, 18*(5), 547–559.

Turnbull, B. W. (1976). The empirical distribution function with arbitrary grouped, censored and truncated data. *Journal of the Royal Statistical Society, 38*, 290–295.

Voinov, V., & Nikulin, M. (1993). *Unbiased estimators and their applications. Univariate case* (Vol. 1). Dordrecht: Kluwer Academic Publishers.

Voinov, V., & Nikulin, M. (1996). *Unbiased estimators and their applications. Multivariate case* (Vol. 2). Dordrecht: Kluwer Academic Publishers.

Voinov, V., Nikulin, M., & Balakrishnan, N. (2013). *Chi-squared goodness of fit tests with applications*. Amsterdam: Academic Press.

Wei, L. J. (1984). Testing goodness-of-fit for the propotional hazards model with censored observations. *Journal of the American Statistical Association, 79*, 649–652.

Wu, H.-D. I. (2004). Effect of ignoring heterogeneity in hazards regression. In M. Nikulin, N. Balakrishnan, M. Mesbah, & N. Limnios (Eds.), *Parametric and semipametric models with applicatiions to reliability, survival analysis, and quality of life* (pp. 239–250). Boston: Birkhauser.

Wu, H.-D. I. (2006). Statistical inference for two-sample and regression models with heterogeneity effects: A collected-sample perspective. In M. Nikulin, D. Commenges, & C. Huber (Eds.), *Probability, statistics and modelling in public health* (pp. 452–465). New York: Springer.

Wu, H.-D. I. (2007). A partial score test for difference among heterogeneous populations. *Journal of Statistical Planning and Inference, 137*, 527–537.

Wu, H.-D. I., Hsieh, F., & Chen, C.-H. (2002). Validation of a heteroscedastic hazards regression model. *Lifetime Data Analysis, 8*, 21–34.

Wu, H.-D. I., & Hsieh, F. (2009). Heterogeneity and varying effect in hazards regression. *Journal of Statistical Planning and Inference, 139*, 4213–4222.

Wulfsohn, M. S., & Tsiatis, A. A. (1997). A joint model for survival and longitudinal data measured with error. *Biometrics, 53*, 330–339.

Yang, S., & Prentice, R. L. (1999). Semiparametric inference in the proportional odds regression model. *Journal of the American Statistical Association, 94*, 125–136.

Ying, Z. (1993). A large sample study of rank estimation for censored regression data. *Annals of Statistics, 21*, 76–99.

Zeng, D., & Lin, D. Y. (2007). Maximum likelihood estimation in semiparametric regression models with censored data. *Journal of the Royal Statistical Society, B69*, 509–564.

Index

A
Aalen's additive risk model, 42
Absence of memory property, 42
Accelerated failure time model, 54
Accelerated life models, 26
Accelerated life regression models, 25
Accelerated life testing, 9
Accelerated stress, 37
Additive accumulation of damage model, 33
Additive hazards (AH) model, 42
Additive–multiplicative hazards (AMH) model, 42
Admissible stress, 25
AFT model, 32
Aging, 9, 109
σ-algebra, 21
Analysis of gastric cancer data, 77
An improvement, 50
At-risk process, 20

B
Baseline cumulative hazard, 69
Baseline hazard rate function, 35
Baseline survival function, 31
Bile duct cancer data, 19
Birnbaum–Saunders model, 15
Breslow estimator, 44, 76

C
Censored data, 20
Censoring processes, 21
Censoring time, 20
Cervical cancer research, 18
Change point model, 64
Changing shape and scale model, 56

Chemo- plus radiotherapy, 77
Chemotherapy, 4, 77
Clinical trials, 1
Compensator, 22
Constant in time stress, 26, 28
Contingency table, 46
Conventional Cox's estimator, 83
Conventional Cox's model, 69
Convex and concave degradation models, 111
Counting process, 22, 68
Covariate, 1, 26
Cox model, 1, 35, 40
Cox-type model with varying coefficients, 65
Crack, 15
Critical threshold, 110
Cross-effect model, 63, 71
Cross-effect of survival functions, 5
Cross-effect phenomena, 5
Cross point, 65
Cumulative distribution function, 10
Cumulative hazard function, 10
Cumulative hazards ratio, 72
Cyclic stress, 15, 28

D
Degradation, 2, 6
Degradation data, 109
Degradation of systems, 109
Degradation path, 111
Degradation process, 25, 109
Degradation-threshold-shock models, 111
Demography, 1
Doob-Meyer decomposition, 22
Dynamic environment, 31

© The Author(s) 2016
M. Nikulin and H.-D.I. Wu, *The Cox Model and Its Applications*,
SpringerBriefs in Statistics, DOI 10.1007/978-3-662-49332-8

E

Econometrics, 1
Empirical distribution, 19
Empirical distribution function, 12
Equipercentile equating method, 31
Equipercentile equation, 32
Equipercentile transfer functional, 32
Explanatory variables, 25
Exponential model, 13
Exponential resource, 30
Exponentiated Weibull model, 16
Extreme value distribution, 59

F

Failure time, 10
Fatigue, 1
Fatigue failure, 15
Filtration, 22
Fleming-Harrington weight function, 83
Flexible models, 32
Flexible regression model, 31
Frailty model, 59
Frailty variable, 59
Full likelihood, 68
Functional delta method, 75

G

Gamma distribution, 14, 62
Gamma frailty model, 62
Gamma model, 14
Gastric cancer data, 2, 93
General degradation path models, 111
Generalized linear PH model, 61
Generalized probit model, 41, 59
Generalized proportional hazards model, 57, 71
Generalized Sedyakin's model, 53
General non-proportional hazards model, 63
Gerontology, 1
Gill-Schumacher test, 82
Gompertz-Makeham model, 13
Goodness-of-fit for the Cox model, 81
Goodness-of-fit problem, 81
Goodness-of-fit test, 95
GPH and SCE models, 84
GPH model, 74
G-resource, 30
G-resource used till the moment t, 30

H

Hazard rate function, 10

H

Hazard ratio, 61
Heteroscedastic hazards regression model, 36
Heteroscedastic Weibull regression, 65
History of failures, 21
Homogeneity effect, 81
Homogeneity hypothesis, 19, 89
Homogeneity test, 81
Hougaard–Aalen model, 72
Hougaard–Aalen model with cross-effects, 72
Hsieh model, 63
Hypertabastic model, 17

I

Instantaneous rate of mortality, 10
Inverse Gaussian distribution, 61
Inverse Gaussian frailty model, 61
Inverse Gaussian model, 15

J

Johansen's decomposition, 68

K

Kalbfleisch and Prentice data, 93
Kaplan-Meier estimator, 23
Karnofsky index, 6, 95
Karnofsky rating, 6
Kong and Slud's test, 50

L

Lack of memory, 13
Left truncated and right-censored data, 96
Left-truncated samples, 22
Length of hospital stay, 2
Lifespan, 1
Lifetime, 10
Likelihood function, 12
Lin and Wei's test, 48
Linear degradation, 111
Linear transformation model, 55
Lin test, 83
Local log partial likelihood, 66
Logistic regression model, 41
Log-linear model, 55
Log-logistic model, 14
Log-logistic survival function, 59
Log-normal family, 14
Log-rank test, 46
Logrank-type statistic, 90
Longevity, 109

Longitudinal data, 110
Lung cancer data, 2, 93
Lung cancer trials, 6

M
Martingale, 23
Maximum likelihood estimator, 12
McKeague and Sasieni model, 43
Median, 3
Method of moments, 23
Mismatch score, 2
Model GM, 39
Model of Lin and Ying, 42
Model with monotone hazard ratio, 59
Modified partial likelihood function, 76
Modified score function, 84
Mortality, 5
Multiple cross-effects model, 78
Multiplicative intensities model, 22

N
Natural degradation process, 10
Nelson–Aalen estimator, 23
Nonparametric estimation, 33
Nonparametric model, 19, 35
Normal stress, 31
Null hypothesis, 87

O
Omnibus test, 82
Ovarian cancer data, 19

P
Parameter of intensity of events, 13
Parametric model, 10, 12, 18, 35
Partial likelihood, 69
Partial likelihood estimation, 43
Partly parametric additive risk model, 43
Performance status, 6
Phenomena of aging, 30
Piantadosi data, 93
Positive stable distribution, 60
Positive stable frailty model, 60
Power generalized Weibull model, 15
Predictable weight processes, 46
Probability density, 10, 16
Progressive stress, 28
Property of absence of memory, 36
Proportional hazards model, 71
Proportional hazards (PH) model, 35

Proportional hazards test, 81
Proportional odds model, 59

R
Radiotherapy, 4
Random stress, 28
Rate of resource using, 32
Rehabilitating stroke, 4
Reliability, 1
Resource, 30
Right-censored data, 20
Right-censored mechanism, 20
Right-censored observations, 4
Robust inference, 47
Robust tests, 46
Robust Wald test, 48
Rule of time-shift, 53

S
Sandwich variance estimator, 47
Scale parameter, 14
Score function, 43, 85
Sedyakin's model, 54
Semi-parametric Cox model, 35
Semi-parametric model, 18
Shape parameter, 14
Sieve approximation, 65, 69
Simple cross-effect model, 63, 71
Simple step stress, 36, 53
Stablein and Koutrouvelis data, 95
Stable index, 60
Standard condition, 25
Standard normal distribution function, 15
Stanford Heart Transplant data, 2, 45
Statistical inference, 25
Step-stress, 26
Stress, 26
Survival analysis, 1
Survival and longitudinal data, 112
Survival data, 63
Survivor function, 24

T
Tampered failure rate, 39
Tampered failure time model, 38
Test for homogeneity, 88
Tests for model validity, 81
The AFT, GPH, LT, frailty, and GLPH models, 53
Transfer functional, 32
Transplant indicators, 2

Two-sample data, 77
Two-sample problem, 88

U
Unimodal, 16, 17

W
Wald-type statistic, 88
Weibull model, 13
Weibull survival function, 59
Weighted log-rank test, 46
Wilcoxon-Peto-Prentice statistic, 92
Wulfsohn and Tsiatis model, 113

Printed in the United States
By Bookmasters